Praise for
Straight Talk about
Psychiatric Medications for Kids

"A Harvard psychiatry professor, researcher, and clinician, [Dr. Wilens] presents a valuable 'insider's' guide to specific disorders (e.g., ADHD, depression, anxiety, autism). Filled with helpful tables and charts, definitions, commonly asked questions, and sources for further information and support, this book should empower parents to become collaborators in their children's care."
—*Library Journal*

"A real 'how-to' for anyone whose child is being treated with medication for psychiatric problems. This book empowers caregivers to manage their children's care more effectively." —**Judith L. Rapoport, MD,**
author of *The Boy Who Couldn't Stop Washing*

"This book—a virtual teaching manual—uses a no-frills approach to providing an affordable wealth of information, a reference/bible that is an excellent supplement to the doctor visit. It is concise, well organized, and very easy to use."
—*NAMI Advocate* **(National Alliance for the Mentally Ill)**

"Readable, thorough, and up-to-date, this book provides cutting-edge information about an important topic. To date, no other book has filled this role. It is a 'must read' for families and educators who want to make sense of the complex issues of when medications may be considered for children and adolescents, and what to expect." —**Henrietta L. Leonard, MD,**
coauthor of *Is It "Just a Phase"?* and *It's Not All in Your Head*

"This volume is unique in that it presents a balanced viewpoint: Although the author clearly states the benefits of appropriate medication in many psychiatric disorders, he just as clearly understands the limitations, potential adverse drug reactions, and familial stresses associated with such an approach....an ongoing theme is the need to build a partnership between the family and clinician in the therapeutic endeavor....The book meets its goals admirably."
—*Science Books & Films*

"Reader-friendly and empathic in tone."
—*Our Children: The National PTA Magazine*

STRAIGHT TALK ABOUT
PSYCHIATRIC MEDICATIONS FOR KIDS

STRAIGHT TALK ABOUT PSYCHIATRIC MEDICATIONS FOR KIDS

Revised Edition

TIMOTHY E. WILENS, MD

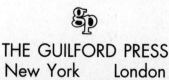

THE GUILFORD PRESS
New York   London

© 2004 Timothy E. Wilens

Published by The Guilford Press
A Division of Guilford Publications, Inc.
72 Spring Street, New York, NY 10012
www.guilford.com

The information in this volume is not intended as a substitute for consultation with healthcare professionals. Each individual's health concerns should be evaluated by a qualified professional.

Printed in the United States of America

This book is printed on acid-free paper.

Last digit is print number: 9 8 7 6 5 4 3 2 1

Library of Congress Cataloging-in-Publication Data

Wilens, Timothy E.
  Straight talk about psychiatric medications for kids / Timothy E. Wilens.—Rev. ed.
    p. cm.
  Includes bibliographical references and index.
  ISBN 1-57230-945-8 (pbk.: alk. paper)—ISBN 1-59385-031-X (hardcover: alk. paper)
  1. Pediatric psychopharmacology—Popular works. I. Title.
  RJ504.7.W54 2004
  618.92′8918—dc22

                                              2004008060

ACKNOWLEDGMENTS

My ability to write this book is a reflection of the environment in which I was raised and practice medicine. One does not simply wake up and find oneself a physician. That process is one that often begins early in life and is nurtured emotionally and intellectually. As you read this book, you will undoubtedly feel the influence of my mother, the liberal social worker, and my father, the conservative businessman-philosopher. I am forever indebted to my family, who have in no small way provided support and confidence to me throughout my life. Their dissatisfaction with the status quo, future-oriented discussions, and intellectual curiosity provided the template on which I operate.

I am grateful to many colleagues who have so willingly shared their experiences with the sundry agents being used in children. I am honored to be part of the Pediatric Psychopharmacology Clinic and Research Program at the Massachusetts General Hospital (MGH) and am grateful to my colleagues for their long-standing support, both of my work in the field and in completing this book. Few professionals have the opportunity and supportive environment available to them to care for patients and conduct clinical research. I am particularly indebted to Dr. Joseph Biederman, Professor of Psychiatry at the Harvard Medical School, who has served as my longtime mentor and whom I and the field of psychiatry greatly admire. His devotion, insight, passion, and thoughtfulness, which have guided the clinical research in this area, have profoundly impacted the lives of psychiatrically impaired children worldwide. I am also deeply appreciative of my close colleague who sits across from me from day to day, Dr. Thomas Spencer, whose friendship, originality, and keen and witty mind have been a great resource in our sharing of the unique clinical and research dilemmas so common in psychiatry.

I also would like to acknowledge the very insightful comments from Chris Benton, who has provided valuable editorial guidance throughout the process of the original and edited versions of *Straight Talk*. I also appreciate the assistance of Dr. Shashank V. Joshi in improving the readability of the book.

One of the greatest honors afforded in our society is being entrusted with the responsibility to care for others as a practitioner of medicine. My respect for my patients and their families is immense and is sprinkled with appreciation for their patience and trust, even after the eighth medication trial has failed. Through our collaborative relationships, I have grown and continue to learn and study the safe and effective use of medications in children. I am also very grateful to the families who have participated in research studies at the MGH and elsewhere to advance our knowledge in pediatric psychopharmacology.

CONTENTS

INTRODUCTION

Should you allow your child to be treated with medication for a mental, emotional, or behavioral problem? If you do, how will you ensure that your child gets the best possible treatment with the least possible risk? How can you be confident that your child has received an accurate diagnosis and that all available avenues of treatment have been considered? What do you need to know to monitor your child's care? If your child is among the estimated 12–22% of American kids—7.5–14 million all together—who suffer from psychiatric disorders, you are facing tough questions like these and many more.

In my 15 years at the Pediatric Psychopharmacology Clinic and Research Program at Massachusetts General Hospital and Harvard Medical School, I have learned that considering medication for a child's psychiatric disorder is one of the most anxiety-producing decisions that many parents ever face, largely because so many questions remain unanswered. The parents I see do not want to be merely sent out the door of my office with a prescription in hand. They want to understand their child's underlying condition and what causes it. They want to learn everything they can about treatments and how helpful each alternative might be. They want to know how much hope they can have that their child's symptoms will improve and their family's well-being will be restored. They want to be effective guardians of their child's psychological health and informed collaborators with their child's mental health practitioners. What they need is straight talk—honest and complete answers to the many complex questions that come up in the course of their child's treatment.

1

This book is an attempt to anticipate and answer all the questions you may have when your child has a mental, emotional, or behavioral problem that could be treated with medication. Since the first edition of this book was published 5 years ago, the field of child psychiatry in general and pediatric pharmacology in particular has seen some notable advances. We have refined our diagnostic skills to better identify bipolar disorder in kids, autistic spectrum illness, anxiety disorders, and the various subtypes of attention-deficit/hyperactivity disorder (ADHD), including its persistence into adulthood. The pharmaceutical industry has come up with new forms of stimulants that make treatment of ADHD easier for children and their parents. We've discovered medications that in very low doses can ease some of the most difficult side effects of psychiatric medications for youngsters. And research into the genetic causes of mental illness and the workings of the brain continues to be vital and fruitful.

Yet, along with new answers have come new questions, which, not surprisingly, join some of the old questions that remain unanswered: What happens to psychiatric disorders in children when they become adults? What are the long-term effects of psychiatric medications on children? Does bipolar disorder really occur in children, and if so, how do we recognize it? Are the subtypes of ADHD accurate reflections of the forms this disorder takes in children? As it did when originally published, this book addresses concerns that are likely to arise when you are just beginning to investigate what may be wrong with your child, all the way through psychiatric evaluation and diagnosis, treatment decisions, and long-term use of medications. The information offered in the following pages is derived from a wealth of scientific literature, ongoing research efforts in which my colleagues and I are engaged, and my own clinical experience. It represents the latest information available at the time of this writing and to my knowledge is still, as was the first edition, the most extensive lay person's book in print on the various medications used to treat children and adolescents with psychiatric disorders. Naturally, information in this field is only growing, making condensation more difficult. Nevertheless, I've made every attempt to keep the information and advice up to date, reflecting some of the most recent literature in the field. In most cases, the revision reflects many of the same tenets as the original publication; yet for some disorders (e.g., bipolar disorder, complicated ADHD) recent advancements have changed the way we conceptualize and treat these conditions, so much of the information here has been revised.

My goal is to offer everything you need to know to make the treatment decisions so important to your child's present and future well-being and that of your family. One of the first lessons I learned as a child psychopharmacologist is that every child and family brings with it unique characteristics and response to treatment. This means that the care of your child will be an ongoing learning experience for you, your child and family, and your child's doctor. It also means that you are a crucial player on this team. You are in a unique position to observe your child, you understand your child better than anyone else, and the information that you can provide about what works and what doesn't, about the problems that arise during treatment and the solutions that work best, is invaluable to the practitioner you have chosen to manage your child's care. Many of our research group's findings and much of what you will read in this book, in fact, has been enriched and expanded by the experiences of parents and children I have had the privilege to work with over the years.

My colleagues in the field of child psychiatry have found that, as time goes on, society in general and parents in particular are less and less willing to leave childhood mental, emotional, and behavioral problems untreated. Many parents have suffered problems similar to those their children are facing and simply wish to spare their children the same impairment. More broadly, however, scientists are discovering increasing evidence that psychiatric disorders affecting children are a serious problem that demands attention, not just developmental phases, adjustment problems, or the effects of poor parenting. Many of these illnesses have a biological basis, meaning in part that the chemical messengers in the brain aren't functioning normally. We know that in numerous situations medications that affect neurochemistry can be exceedingly useful in reducing symptoms and restoring children's ability to function well. For all these reasons, pharmacological treatment is an option for parents whose children have psychiatric disorders.

That does not mean, of course, that it is the only option. Psychiatric disorders in children can be complicated to diagnose and complicated to treat. Often the best solution for a given child is a combination of psychotherapy and pharmacology, and sometimes more than one treatment in each category produces the greatest improvement. Frequently only trial and error will tell what works best for your child. This book is by no means an advertisement for psychiatric medications, and I will frankly tell you what I know about adverse effects, limitations, and other problems related to the use of these drugs along with the success stories I have witnessed. This book will supply the facts about common psychiatric disorders affecting children and the currently accepted treatments for them, with up-to-date details on the medications among those treatments. You and your child's practitioner will supply the other half of the equation—an understanding of your child—and the two of you will collaborate on a treatment scheme. Throughout this revised edition, in fact, I will point out the expanded role of the parents in a child's mental health care. Since this book's original publication, it has become increasingly important that a child's parent take on the management of the entire mental health care process, from supervising the child's evaluation to monitoring treatment, managing the child's emotions, and coordinating the efforts of the mental health and educational team. The more facts you have at your disposal, the more effective the parent–practitioner collaboration becomes, the more fruitful the dialogue between you, and the more hope you offer your child. Hopefully you will find the information you seek in the following three sections.

Part I, "What Every Parent Should Know about Psychiatric Medications for Children," is the best place to begin if you need an overview of the issues involved in the medicating process or you have fundamental questions about that process. Part I addresses common concerns in the order in which you will probably encounter them, from the preliminaries to the evaluation and diagnosis of your child, to the creation of a treatment plan and your child's ongoing care. Part I is presented in question-and-answer format. Read it in its entirety or flip through until you spot the questions that have been on your mind (or use the index to find specific answers you need). The answers include illustrative examples from my own practice (either composites or well disguised to protect the privacy of patients and their families). Interspersed throughout Part I are boxed definitions of terms you're likely to hear often from your child's mental health practitioners. In this revised edition I've added questions and answers on issues that have received great attention or to which more information has recently become available over the past few years, with a special focus on helping you become the best manager of your child's diagnosis and treatment that you can be—a collection of tasks that becomes more important with every passing year.

Part II, "Common Childhood Psychiatric Disorders," provides information on common symptoms, biology, causes, course (what happens to the disorder with time), and other conditions that often accompany the disorder for the major emotional and behavioral disorders that we see in children and adolescents. Each chapter ends with a review of the major medications and other interventions used in treatment. Diagnostic criteria and methods are always being reviewed and revised to reflect new research and clinical findings, and in this edition you'll discover what we've recently learned about bipolar disorder, Asperger syndrome, ADHD, and other disorders for which new information has come to light. These disorders are grouped by related symptoms or the problems associated with them. If your child has been diagnosed with a particular condition and you do not know which heading it falls under, check the index.

Part III, "The Psychotropic Medications," offers detailed descriptions of the major classes of medications used to treat psychiatric disorders in kids. Included are the common uses of the medications, areas of the brain and neurotransmitters affected by the medications, available preparations and strengths, dosing information, safe combinations with other agents, and extensive details on side effects. Questions and answers on typical concerns and problems raised by parents are featured throughout these chapters. Here, as in Parts I and II, I've updated the chapters to provide the latest information on new medications, new forms of older medications, and recent findings about the administration and effectiveness of these agents in children and teenagers. In some cases, major sections have been rewritten and the order of use of certain classes of medications has been changed drastically, reflecting new data on what works best and longer-term safety issues associated with specific classes of medication.

In discussing medications, I refer to each drug by its most commonly used name. In some cases this is the brand name, which is capitalized (e.g., Prozac or Ritalin). In other cases this is the generic name, which appears in lowercase letters (e.g., desipramine). A list of medications and their generic and brand names, as well as their suggested preparation and strengths, is available in the Appendix (pp. 265–269).

In discussing mental health professionals, I use various terms, from *doctor* to *practitioner* to *clinician* and other terms. Who provides what type of care for your child will vary, depending on your location, your health care plan, and the availability of specialists. I may refer to your child's pediatrician or prescribing physician when discussing a service that this particular professional is likely to offer, but in other cases, when you see the term *doctor,* please understand that it means the person responsible for the relevant facet of your child's care.

Likewise, I use the term *child* to mean anyone who has not yet reached adulthood. Where the subject applies exclusively to adolescents or younger children, I will state that.

At the back of the book you'll find information on where to go for more information and for the support that many parents find helpful in meeting the challenges of raising a child with a mental, behavioral, or emotional problem. If you don't find what you need from any of these sources, don't forget the resources you already have—not only your child's prescriber, but all the other health care professionals at your disposal, from psychotherapists to nurse practitioners, from social workers to nurses, from your child's pediatrician to your family practitioner. Straight questions from you are the best way to get straight answers.

PART I

What Every Parent Should Know about Psychiatric Medications for Children

When your child has a psychiatric problem for which medication may be prescribed, a thousand questions beg to be answered. Parents come to me with an urgently felt need for information—and often more than a little anxiety as well. In this section, I've compiled the questions that usually come up—in my office as well as at the talks I give about four times a month for professional and parent support groups across the United States, the United Kingdom, and Europe—with the most current, most complete answers that can be given in a book meant to speak to a broad cross-section of parents.

As is stressed throughout the book, you are a key player in your child's mental health care. To fill that role optimally, you need to stay as well informed as you can about your child's problem and the treatments available for it. This involves asking the right questions as well as getting reliable answers. I hope the following questions, posed by hundreds of caring, concerned parents before you, will get you thinking as a proactive collaborator in the care of your child. And I hope the answers will give you some of the comfort and reassurance that knowledge provides. Always remember, though, that your child's situation is unique. The right answers for your son or daughter will always come mainly from the cooperative efforts of you and the qualified professionals you have chosen to care for your child. The importance of your participation in this process cannot be overstated. With managed care and overtaxed practitioners, a labyrinth of legal rights to navigate at school and elsewhere, and the day-to-day challenges of running a household when one (or more) of the children in the family has mental, emotional, or behavioral problems, keeping things operating smoothly can be really tough—and more crucial than ever before. This book concentrates mainly on the use of medications in treating psychiatric disorders in young people, but a wealth of sources is available to help you with the many other jobs you've been handed. I've added to the Resources section at the back of the book, so you know where to find them.

The following questions and answers have been divided into four groups, based on when in the diagnosis and treatment process they usually arise. Questions asked by parents who are just considering seeking help for their child come first. Next are questions and answers for those currently involved in the evaluation process. The third section addresses questions about the diagnosis and the treatment proposal that emerge from the evaluation. The last section addresses issues that come up when a child is already being treated with medications for a psychiatric or psychological disorder. Read all of Part I for an overview or turn to the individual sections and questions within them as needed. Either way, I hope you will find what you need to know. If not, please ask your child's practitioners—that's what they are there for.

CHAPTER 1

THE PRELIMINARIES
Building a Foundation of Knowledge

It is never easy to face the fact that your child may need help for a mental, emotional, or behavioral problem. A tough situation becomes harder when, like most parents, you know little about the subject of childhood psychiatric disorders and their treatment. It gets even more difficult when you're plagued by the misconceptions and myths that abound.

Perhaps you've just consulted your child's pediatrician because your son or daughter has been behaving differently, and the doctor has told you that he or she suspects a certain disorder is present for which medication is usually the recommended treatment. Or you may be wondering if medication could help your child now that a long-standing problem is worsening and no longer manageable by other means. Maybe you're just beginning to believe something might be wrong with your child, and what you've read about similar problems has left you confused and a little alarmed. You're not alone. More and more people—parents and professionals alike—are considering medication as a viable option for treating many psychiatric problems in children. The field may not be as young as it was when this book first came out, but new myths and misconceptions seem to arise to fill the void left by discarded ones, and of course we still have a lot to learn. The result is that numerous gaps in our collective understanding remain. At this point, parents want to know everything from "Why is medication necessary?" and "Isn't there any other treatment?" to "What will happen if we just wait and watch?" and "How do we know drugs designated for this purpose are safe?" If you are at this stage with your child, the following background should help you decide whether to go ahead and have your child evaluated for possible medical treatment.

What makes the doctor think my child needs medication?

There is no simple answer to why any child may need medications for a psychiatric or psychological problem. Each child's situation is unique, complex, and constantly evolving. Any decision regarding the child's care and treatment should be the result of a thorough evaluation of the many factors involved and a thoughtful consideration of all the alternative solutions available. As I hope to reinforce throughout this book, however, you have an absolute right to seek a satisfactory explanation for any decision about your child's case *from the doctor who has made that decision.* Never be afraid to ask. You should have a good grasp of the conclusions your child's doctor has reached and the rationale that led the doctor to the recommendation before your child embarks on any form of treatment. In fact the entire evaluation, diagnosis, and treatment process should be a collaborative effort between you and your child's health care providers. To broach the subject with your child's doctor, try saying something like "I'm trying to understand your decision-making process. Can you walk me through it?"

Whether your child needs medication depends on the problem, its causes, and its effects on your child's life. Some mental and emotional disturbances are treated successfully with psychotherapy. Others are treated most effectively with a combination of psychotherapy and pharmacology or just medication alone. Typically, a doctor may consider medication based on the belief that the child's problem has a medical cause, or etiology (it's not just "all in the kid's head"), especially one that usually worsens with time or with stresses in the child's life. In cases like this, the child may seem perfectly healthy physically even though the cause of the problem originates in the body. Such medical conditions are frequently unlikely to go away on their own, and the child's symptoms may very well get worse if ignored. Many of the childhood psychiatric conditions for which medication has been used over the past decade fit this description. Attention-deficit/hyperactivity disorder (ADHD) is one example that many parents have read about. Scientists now believe that the impulsivity, short attention span, and other symptoms associated with ADHD are caused by a specific dysfunction in the brain that often is inherited. How severely impaired the child is by the ADHD, however, depends on the severity of the ADHD and on environmental factors such as whether the child's parents and teachers take the child's disability into account in rearing and educating the child. A child whose disability is ignored is likely to suffer academically and socially. In turn, these experiences tend to aggravate the symptoms of ADHD and may even spawn additional problems, such as defiant, destructive behavior. So, if your child's condition is causing even moderate distress and is pervasive, the doctor may have good reason to consider medication management.

> **dysfunction:** The state of not working properly.
>
> **etiology:** The biological or psychological cause of a disorder. The actual disturbances in the body organs or brain causing the disorder are called the pathophysiology.
>
> **pervasive:** Occurring more often than not, in many settings, and for more than a few months.

Like many other psychological disorders, ADHD starts with a problem in the body (the brain), but its whole profile in any one child is formed by a number of interwoven factors. To decide whether medication might be an appropriate treatment for your child's problem, the doctor must take all these ingredients into account. Each human being carries a unique set of experiences and vulnerabilities that combine to make the person more or less susceptible to psychiatric disorders. Some of these factors are environmental (people, events, and stressors in the child's surroundings), some biological (genetic), and most a complex interplay of the two. Depression is a common example in children, with an inherited predisposition often triggered by some external event, such as loss of a loved one.

To diagnose the problem and treat it wisely, the doctor has to understand these factors as thoroughly as possible. Before I could treat 12-year-old Joy, for example, I had to find out not only that she had remained withdrawn, apathetic, and listless for months following her dog's death but also that her mother had been treated for long-standing depression. A tendency toward depression that she may have inherited from her mother was activated by the trauma of losing her beloved pet. In turn, one symptom of depression, Joy's withdrawal from family and friends, increased the environmental impact on her psychological health by removing needed support. This in turn made her depression worse. (I won't go into the details here, but most recent psychiatric research suggests that these environmental factors can cause biological and neurological changes that may appear to be inborn biological abnormalities.

These complexities present a formidable diagnostic and treatment task that demands input from those who know the child best—the child's parents. Your insight can head the doctor in the right treatment direction, shortening what can be a somewhat lengthy process of trial and error. In fact your child's doctor may suggest psychopharmacological treatment—treatment with drugs designed to treat psychiatric problems—after getting less-than-satisfactory results from other forms of treatment. Although the efficacy of drugs is becoming more widely known, psychotherapy is often the first-line treatment for mental, emotional, and behavioral problems in both children and adults. However, there has been a shift in categorically recommending psychotherapy as first line for all psychiatric disorders in children and adults. As you may already know if you were initially referred to a psychologist by your child's pediatrician or teacher, various types of psychotherapy have been developed in this burgeoning field. If your child is already seeing a therapist without noticeable improvement, the therapist may have referred you to a psychiatrist (or back to your pediatrician) for further evaluation. Many children, for example, worry excessively after their parents' divorce. But if a child continues worrying excessively for more than a year despite counseling, other treatments, including pharmacotherapy, may be worth considering. The practitioner may conclude that psychotherapy alone is not sufficient in your child's particular situation. Or the doctor may be aware, from personal clinical experience or psychiatric literature, that medication has been shown to work more effectively for your child's disorder than psychotherapy alone.

If a doctor suggests medication for your child, it is not necessarily cause for alarm. With most health problems, we tend to believe that the need for medical treatment—as opposed to lifestyle changes or no treatment at all—is a sign that the problem is relatively severe. This is not always the case with psychiatric disorders. Sometimes a medication offers the straightforward solution to the child's problem because some agent specifically targets the medical cause of the disorder. In ADHD, for example, medicines bring improvement in a way that no other form of treatment alone has been able to do. Likewise, bipolar disorder in children generally cannot be managed without a mood-stabilizing medication. Thus, medication may be a powerful mechanism to help alleviate your child's problem, either as a single treatment or in concert with psychotherapy.

A good way to approach the issue of medications for your child is to stay as open-minded as you can. Objective information gathering will help you make an informed decision. Try not to let fear of the unknown sway you before you tap all the sources available to increase your understanding. Later in this section, I'll go into more detail about when medication generally benefits children and how it works. (And for more specific information, consult the chapters in Parts II and III that cover your child's disorder, if it has already been diagnosed, or the medication that is being recommended, if you've already had such recommendations from the doctor.) For now, view medication as one option for helping your child. Be prepared to balance its benefits against both the risks of the medication itself and the risks of *not* using medication (taking a "wait-and-see" approach).

If my child takes medications, everyone—teachers, babysitters, relatives, friends—will know something is really wrong. Won't this make things even harder for my son?

Again, remember that the need for medication is not necessarily a sign of severity. If anyone who knows about your son's treatment expresses undue alarm about it, share the information you have gathered about medication's role in treating this type of problem. Knowing that medication is one of the treatments of choice for many childhood psychiatric disorders often reassures and prevents people from overreacting in ways that will make your son self-conscious. In general, though, you should probably discuss your child's disorder only on a need-to-know basis. Before you air any aspect of the subject, ask yourself whether this person needs the information to protect your child's well-being. If not, treat the information as private and confidential: Keep it to yourself. (Note, too, that extended-release forms of the stimulants used to treat ADHD have recently become available, meaning in many cases that children no longer have to "announce" their problem through regular trips to the nurse's office at school. See pages 210–212 for more information.)

Sadly, there are people who will use their knowledge of your son's treatment as a weapon ("*Oh,* Johnny's on medication—*no wonder* he's so impossible"). There are also many people today who still harbor misconceptions about psychiatric disorders. It is your job to protect your child from the myths and prejudices that range from labeling your child as "feeble-minded" to portraying him as "crazy." Share what you have learned, but also examine your own attitudes.

Many parents seem to come to grips with medical disorders such as diabetes or seizures but have great difficulty accepting emotional and behavioral problems in children. Are you among those who hold an irrational fear of mental illness or who look down on those with psychiatric disorders? Defensiveness about your child's condition may stem from your own lingering doubts. Try to remember that you may very well be dealing with just another type of medical problem. Emerging findings suggest that the bulk of emotional, cognitive, and behavioral disorders are caused by subtle chemical differences in the brains of children. The medications that are prescribed normalize the transmission of these chemical signals and thus reduce the child's symptoms.

> **disorder:** A cluster of symptoms and objective findings that, grouped together, are related to a specific problem.
>
> **symptom:** A manifestation of a disorder. Cough and fever are symptoms of pneumonia; sadness and lack of appetite are symptoms of depression.

Passing this information on to others can go a long way toward erasing the stigma surrounding psychiatric disorders, especially because it eliminates the need to assign blame for the child's condition. Any anxiety you may be feeling about your child's problem can be exaggerated by the conventional notion that mental and emotional disturbances are caused solely by the way you are raising your child. Parents of my patients often seem to encounter this bias at their child's school. Despite the plethora of teachers, guidance counselors, and other school staff who understand and empathize with families who are struggling with psychiatric problems, there always seem to be a vocal few who are quick to point the finger of blame. If you run into this attitude, remember that school personnel do not live with your family and often cannot fully appreciate the scope of the situation. You may be tagged as "the nervous type" because your child's behavior is not so disruptive in the relative structure of the school setting. Or you may be considered irresponsible if you express little concern about behavior problems you don't see at home—such as the peer problems and academic problems that tend to appear mainly at school.

Here, too, the solution is education. Explain to those at your child's school and elsewhere what you have learned about the biological causes of the child's disorder. Remind those who remain skeptical that it wasn't until recently that scientists discovered a biological basis for alcoholism and drug addiction. We don't blame others for causing someone's alcoholism today, and we should not blame parents or anyone else for causing a child's psychiatric disorder. *Your child's problem is not necessarily your fault.*

Nor is it your child's fault. Make sure your child does not view the disorder as some sort of personal failing or weakness. Explain, in understandable terms that take the child's age into account, that the child has a problem that he can't help having. (For fairness and simplicity's sake, I will alternate between male and female pronouns.) Say that this problem is largely physical in the same way Aunt Alice's asthma is physical or Daddy's high blood pressure is physical. If medication is a possibility, tell your child that it's no different from the inhaler that helps Aunt Alice breathe or the pills that keep Daddy's blood pressure under control. Also assure the child that many other kids take medications without anyone else knowing about it—maybe including some of your son's or daughter's friends. You may have to offer these reassurances repeatedly over a long period if this problem has been emerging and causing distress gradually over time.

What options do we have besides medication?

The answer depends on which disorder your child has. Check the chapter in Part II that addresses your child's problem for more specific information on the standard treatment choices. Generally, though, the options break down into psychotherapy and pharmacotherapy, and often a combination of the two proves most effective. There is a bewildering array of psychotherapies available today. To unravel the possibilities, you might need to ask your doctor, your friends, or others who have some firsthand experience about the options.

> **psychotherapy**: An umbrella term that covers the broad range of "talking" therapies.
>
> **pharmacotherapy**: Treatment of a condition using medications.

Because psychiatric disorders almost invariably affect a child's behavior, a variety of interventions that target behavior are commonly used. Using clinically proven methods, therapists can help children with bipolar disorder (manic–depression) and ADHD control their impulsivity, help those with Tourette's disorder lessen their disruptive verbalizing, and teach teenagers with eating disorders to regain the proper perspective on the role of food in their lives. Behavioral and cognitive therapies can alleviate the primary symptoms of some psychiatric disorders (such as hair pulling [trichotillomania] and obsessive–compulsive disorder) and in other cases can address behavioral problems that are an offshoot of the disorder. For example, a child with ADHD can be taught to pause before acting on an impulse; one who has oppositional defiant disorder can learn to comply rather than defy when the parents habitually punctuate positive behavior and ignore negative behavior. Most important is understanding what any therapy chosen for your child can be expected to change in a given disorder. Recent research is beginning to show, for example, that a type of cognitive behavioral therapy has the same beneficial effects on neurotransmitters as the use of medication. But in the case of bipolar disorder, behavioral interventions cannot cure the child of the biological tendency toward mood swings, even though it may be able to help her learn to recognize the signs of mood changes and what actions to take when she does experience them.

> **neurotransmitters**: Chemical messengers that are the main communications link' between nerve cells.

Other forms of therapy for the child include interpersonal and dynamic-oriented therapies, social skills training, family therapy, peer interventions, relaxation training, and many others. These all offer different benefits and at times can address some of the core issues of mental disorders but often are aimed at the secondary effects. For example, Jason, who has ADHD, has no friends at school and fights with his siblings at home. He benefited from social skills training, peer group interventions, as well as family therapy. Often primary care providers will not advise that a child undergo numerous types of therapy all at once.

Try to find out from your child's mental health provider which issues have a high priority and which form of counseling if any might be of greatest help right now.

How aggressively your child is treated will depend largely on the urgency of improving the child's condition. When the child is a danger to herself or others, or the child or family is suffering greatly from the child's disorder, you will not want to take a wait-and-see attitude. On the other hand, parents and the doctor should not rush into a treatment recommendation without sensitivity to the child's possible reactions. With an oppositional, depressed teenager, for example, it might be crucial to develop a trusting relationship with a practitioner before trying medication. To push medication immediately could very well cause the child to reject current care and compromise any future possibility for intervention.

Ask the doctor to help you weigh the risks of medication treatment against the risks of delaying the treatment. Ask questions like "What do you think would happen if we tried psychotherapy first?" and "Can you list the major pros and cons of starting medication right away?"

If we're patient, won't the problem just go away as my child gets older?

Whereas some behavioral, cognitive, and emotional problems improve with the child's development, others may persist. Depression and generalized anxiety, for instance, do not seem to disappear as the child ages; they merely manifest themselves in different ways. Depression, for example, may appear as irritability, withdrawal, and lack of interest (apathy) in younger kids, while depressed teenagers may complain of sadness, lack of energy, social problems, and suicidal thoughts. One recent longitudinal study of bipolar disorder showed that there is a high rate of remission and relapse in kids with this diagnosis but a low rate of true cures. You'll find more on this subject in the chapters on specific disorders in Part II, and your child's mental health care providers can tell you what the future may hold for your child.

> **cognitive:** Related to thinking or knowing.
>
> **longitudinal:** Related to what happens to a disorder over time.

Even with disorders that sometimes go into remission with maturity, though, it is a mistake to ignore the problem in the expectation that it will just go away. It is always difficult to predict *when* a disorder will abate, and in the meantime, doing nothing can damage your child. The reports of many adults confirm what we intuitively know: Neglecting treatment in a child with behavioral and emotional problems may lead to serious future problems. We simply do not know when those scars develop but speculate that it is an ongoing process over years born of underachievement, demoralization, lack of confidence, and poor self-esteem. Eight-year-old Justin, for example, who has a severe anxiety disorder (excessive worrying), began avoiding social situations despite wanting friends. Intensive treatment of his condition with behavioral modification and Tranxene reduced his anxiety substantially, allowed him to socialize normally, and improved his self-esteem and confidence greatly. Clearly, if your child is achieving below her potential and seems discouraged and down on herself, you should take action, whether that means seeking an initial psychiatric evaluation, switching from psychotherapy alone to drug or combined therapy, or trying a new medication regimen. Other troubling signs include loss of interest in learning, long-standing displeasure, and poor social skills and relationships for the child's age.

When my brother heard that our pediatrician thinks Jenny is suffering from depression, he started telling me about his symptoms, which are so different that I started to have doubts about what's wrong with Jenny. Should I question the pediatrician?

Certainly you should always ask questions when you have doubts or concerns about anything your child's doctor tells you. You may also want to have your pediatrician refer you to a mental health specialist so you can be sure you know everything you need to know about your daughter's condition. But don't assume that differences between Jenny's symptoms and your adult brother's symptoms mean the pediatrician is wrong. There is growing evidence in the scientific literature that psychiatric disorders starting in childhood are often somewhat different from those in adulthood. Juvenile-onset bipolar disorder, for one, often features intertwined depression and mania rather than the more typically distinct phases of either depression or mania seen in the adult-onset form. It is important to understand these distinctions because they may explain why a child's response to medications sometimes differs from the adult responses with which you may already be familiar. For developmental reasons, a child with a particular disorder may have different symptoms from an adult with the disorder of the same name. The course may differ as well. As a general rule, with notable exceptions, psychiatric disorders that begin in early childhood often are more severe, tend to be chronic (sustained), and often run in families.

> **course:** What happens to a condition over time.

Current thinking indicates that a sizable number of children who have childhood disorders have genetic vulnerabilities to the disorder that were passed on by their parents and grandparents. These vulnerabilities may be turned on spontaneously or by an environmental problem or stressor. In the case of 7-year-old Molly—whose parents both suffered from depression—feelings of sadness, isolation, and withdrawal began following the death of her grandmother, continued for 4 months, and were accompanied by school and social difficulties. After a month of psychotherapy, Molly's depression was reduced dramatically. We suspected that the stress of losing her grandmother had triggered in Molly a depression stemming from a biological predisposition toward depression inherited from her parents.

As a parent, you've witnessed the differences between medical illnesses in children and those in adults. You may also be aware of the differences in common chronic diseases like diabetes and rheumatoid arthritis. Compared to adult-onset diabetes, juvenile-onset diabetes mellitus (type I) requires insulin injections, does not appear to be inherited (genetic), and tends to be more severe. Juvenile rheumatoid arthritis is very different from the adult version in the joint regions affected, genetic vulnerabilities, and overall course. It should be no surprise, then, that psychiatric disorders that begin in childhood can also look quite different from those that begin in adulthood. Very recent work on bipolar disorder (manic–depression) in children and adolescents, for example, indicates that children may have severe symptoms of both mania ("high") and depression at the same time for extended periods. In contrast, adults more typically have distinct cycles of mania and then depression and often have periods of normal mood. At least half of children with bipolar disorder, not surprisingly, have a close relative with the same disorder.

Unfortunately, we are just beginning to understand how psychiatric disorders in childhood will evolve over time and into adulthood. Whereas there is relatively solid evidence that conduct disorder often progresses to the antisocial personality disorder of adulthood (the prognosis is worse with early onset, under age 10, than when conduct disorder begins after age 10), less is known about the adult fate of depressed children. Many adults with anxiety disorders report that their problems began when they were younger, but the exact path of anxiety from childhood to adulthood remains unclear. Of interest, some new studies indicate that infants with a type of temperament (hard-wired personality traits) known as behavioral inhibition may be predisposed to developing more severe anxiety problems or shyness as children.

The good news is that a number of disorders that affect children appear to get better, to some degree, with time. Younger children appear to grow out of severe anxiety related to separation from their parents or primary caregivers with time. Kids with oppositionality also commonly out-grow their argumentative and annoying features as young adults. Another common example is ADHD, which is thought to disappear (remit) by adulthood in roughly half of the children affected, particularly the hyperactivity symptoms of the disorder. Recent information is telling us that, while the hyperactive and impulsive symptoms of ADHD improve largely in adolescence, the prominent attentional deficits continue into adulthood, still causing problems in many areas of life. The field is still trying to figure out the best way to diagnose adults with ADHD.

Another feature of childhood psychiatric problems is that many young people have two or three different disorders simultaneously. Whether these disorders just happen to run together, as is the case for some children with bipolar disorder and ADHD, or one disorder leads to another, as may happen in children with long-standing obsessive–compulsive disorder who develop depressive symptoms because of demoralization, is unclear. Whatever the suspected cause, the occurrence of two or more disorders together is called comorbidity. A child with depression and anxiety, for example, would be said to have comorbid anxiety and depression, without any causality being implied.

It is important to keep the possibility of comorbidity in mind because, in many children, new symptoms or problems surface once the diagnosed disorder is treated successfully. Rather than just writing this off to the environment or, worse, a dysfunctional family that will not "let" the child get better, it is medically sound to evaluate the child for the presence of another disorder. Fourteen-year-old Mike's severe obsessionality was greatly reduced when his obsessive–compulsive disorder was treated with 200 mg of Zoloft a day, along with *cognitive behavioral therapy,* but his academic problems continued. As it turned out, those problems were caused by inattention and distractibility related to ADHD, which had gone undiagnosed because of the severity of his obsessive–compulsive condition. Additional stimulant treatment for the ADHD proved very effective.

If you suspect that your child has more than one problem, be prepared to enumerate all the specific symptoms with the practitioner who ends up doing the evaluation. By carefully asking questions about the more common behavioral and emotional disorders in children, your child's doctor can disentangle the overlap of symptoms and make reasonable sense of your child's condition. If a child has rather clear-cut depression, for instance, the presence of other common disorders such as anxiety, ADHD, and substance abuse should be considered. Some commonly co-occurring conditions include depression and anxiety, substance abuse and depression, ADHD and anxiety, bipolar disorder and ADHD, Tourette's disorder and ADHD, and anorexia and obsessive–compulsive disorder.

> **substance abuse:** A pattern of misuse of drugs or alcohol generally resulting in interpersonal, occupational, legal, or medical problems.

If drugs work so well in treating children with mental and emotional problems, why do I hear such conflicting reports about them?

Conflicting reports abound mainly because child psychopharmacology is still a relatively new science. You'll hear many more firm conclusions on the subject as time goes on, because so much information is being gathered in clinics and research labs right now, but significant developments have been a long time in coming. Psychoactive substances have been a standard psychiatric treatment for adults for only about 50 years; for children, only about 20. The realization that drugs could benefit children with emotional and behavioral disorders is a fascinating example of how separate branches of science—along with a few fortuitous accidents—can intersect to produce a groundbreaking discovery.

> **psychoactive:** Affecting the central nervous system, resulting in changes in thinking, behavior, or emotion. Synonymous with *psychotropic* and *psychopharmacological.*

As more and more information on brain biochemistry and structure suggested that psychiatric disorders had a biological cause, new and different medications were developed and tested, and further biological studies were undertaken. The 1990s, "the decade of the brain," saw a near revolution in thinking about children's psychiatric disorders. Not long before that, children's emotional and behavioral problems were believed to be rooted entirely in disturbed parenting. But the findings of genetics, neurobiology, and brain imaging studies began to lead mental health and other medical practitioners toward an interactional model. Individuals are now viewed as biological beings interacting with the environment, with each factor influencing the others. This perspective has completely transformed psychiatric views of cause and effect. Now a so-called neurotic child is more likely to be viewed as having a nervous temperament (biology) that induces those around her to be overprotective (environment) than as a child whose overprotective parents have caused her to become "neurotic." Parents were once categorically blamed for the lack of interaction with the environment that characterized autism, but now autism is known to be caused by biologically based abnormalities in the brain. Similarly, ADHD, Tourette's disorder, obsessive–compulsive disorder, and mood disorders have been found to run in families. In fact, while you are reading this, scientists are working to isolate the genes responsible for the different disorders and to develop replacement therapy to correct, at a chromosomal level, the neurochemical disturbances underlying specific conditions.

> **neurobiology**: The basic science underpinning nerves and the nervous system.
>
> **neurochemical**: Referring to the elemental makeup of the messengers of the nervous system.
>
> **neuropsychological**: Related to the interface between brain functioning and thinking processes (perception, processing, and problem solving). Generally refers to the interaction of brain functioning with the process of thinking and vice versa.

You'll be exposed to such developments as the research advances. For now, though, news is sporadic for two reasons: The press hesitates to disseminate information on medication treatments that have not completed the lengthy process of Food and Drug Administration (FDA) approval, and parents are protective of their children's privacy. As you will learn in Parts II and III, your child's doctor may view a certain drug as standard treatment for a particular childhood disorder despite lack of FDA approval for its use in children because a wealth of clinical evidence has been amassed in its favor. By late 2003, many of the medications that had not yet been approved for anyone other than adults when this book was first published had been approved for use in adolescents or even children. Most of the selective serotonin reuptake inhibitors (SSRIs), for example, are now approved for use in adolescents with a variety of conditions, notably obsessive–compulsive disorder. And much more research is being done, thanks to some important federal regulations. One example is the pediatric exclusivity rule (2002), which pressures pharmaceutical companies to evaluate those medications that may be used in children prior to receiving FDA approval for pediatric use. This rule has resulted in many more studies of how medications work and how they are metabolized in children.

If child psychopharmacology is so new, how do we know the medications are safe?

As long as your child takes the medication as prescribed, psychotropic medications are very safe. Many agents listed in this book have been used in children for over two decades with a solid track record. Some, such as the amphetamine preparations, have been used with children since the 1930s. Specific medications, including Ritalin, amphetamines, Tegretol, Depakote, Cylert, desipramine, imipramine, and clonidine, have been known to produce rare severe side effects, so children taking these drugs are monitored closely by the prescriber. Also, we know that the anti-psychotics (Haldol, Stelazine, Trilafon, Mellaril, Thorazine, and others in this family) can cause abnormal muscle movements, called *tardive dyskinesia*, in a small group of kids exposed to these agents for years, so the subtle effects of long-term medication use need to be monitored as well. Of interest, Ritalin and Prozac, medications that some parents view as the most dangerous because of adverse media commentary, turn out to be among the safest being used in children (and adults)!

> **psychopharmacology:** The study of compounds that affect the central nervous system, resulting in changes in thinking, behavior, or emotion.
>
> **psychotropics:** Agents that affect the central nervous system, resulting in changes in thinking, behavior, or emotion. Synonymous with *psychopharmacological* and *psychoactive agents.*
>
> **compound:** A pharmacologically active agent. Synonymous with *medication, drug,* and *agent.*

Because the use of most psychotropic drugs in children is relatively recent, many of these agents have not yet gained FDA approval for pediatric use. Though the confidence that our stringent regulatory process instills has great value, lack of FDA approval does not automatically mean a drug *is* unsafe for psychiatric use in children. By and large all of the medications used by child psychopharmacologists have FDA-approved indications, but they may be approved for conditions or age groups other than the particular condition or age group in question (antiepileptic drugs, antihypertensives, etc.). In many cases, in fact, unapproved drugs have a wealth of clinical evidence to back up their safety and effectiveness; see page 94 for details. We should also be seeing much more safety data in the coming years. In a major step toward recognizing pharmacology as treatment for children with psychiatric disorders, Congress recently passed legislation requiring American drug manufacturers to study medications in children with the potential use in youth before the drug can gain FDA approval for use in adults.

In the meantime, there is no doubt that the greatest danger of medications is an overdose. Although children with certain disorders such as depression are at risk for harming themselves, the bulk of lethal overdoses are accidental and occur in family members or friends, such as when a younger sibling thinks the medication is candy. It is important to remember that medications that are safe in daily administration can be very dangerous in overdose. That is why you have to designate a special storage place (locked cabinet) and policy for your child's medication if drugs become a part of his treatment regimen. And, remember: Parents or legal guardians—not the child—should be responsible at all times for the medications.

What about all of the press on the use of medications in younger kids?

Recently considerable concern has been raised in the media about the use of psychotropic medications in kids younger than 6 years of age. This controversy arose after a highly cited report was published showing a marked increase in the use of medications in this age group over the past 5 years. What emerged was hysteria about why we are "unnecessarily drugging" our kids.

In reality, we are identifying problems earlier and treating them more intensively. There is a great deal of evidence indicating that the earlier a problem emerges in childhood, the more serious and impairing the problem may be. In addition, disorders that start in early childhood often have a strong biological component. Few in medicine would advocate that severe problems be left untreated without an intervention. For example, no one would consider allowing a preschooler with another brain-based disorder, such as seizures, to go untreated. It is becoming clear to researchers in mental health and well known to clinicians that the earlier we intervene and treat problems in kids, the better off youth do as they grow up (e.g., improved self-esteem, less substance abuse). This is the principle by which we operate when considering medicating a younger child. The most common problems we identify and treat with medication include ADHD (characterized by excessive and often dangerous hyperactivity and impulsive behavior), severe moodiness, and incapacitating anxiety. Although family- and behavioral-based therapies are typically suggested initially, these interventions may not be enough to help resolve or treat the problems in some children. In these cases, not only does the child suffer and fall greatly behind in socialization and academics, but the child's family may be victimized by the child's behaviors, such as violent outbursts. Unfortunately, deep-rooted animosity between siblings can solidify to the degree that these youths brutalize their brothers and sisters despite their love for them.

There is no question that we are using medications that have not been extensively tested in preschoolers. However, for the most common problems identified among preschoolers, the field does have some data available, and more studies are currently under way. For example, there have been seven well-controlled studies and there is one large study under way on the use of Ritalin in preschoolers that demonstrate both improvement and the occurrence of predictable side effects. We use ADHD medications such as clonidine or guanfacine to treat excessive hyperactivity and impulsivity, in part, because they are well tolerated without the appetite or sleep side effects, issues of great concern in this age group. We also use antidepressants for kids with severe anxiety, obsessivness, or depression, as well as anticonvulsants to reduce preschoolers' mood swings or aggression. In fact, some specific psychotropics in the stimulant and antipsychotic classes are, indeed, FDA-approved for use for behavioral problems in kids 3 years and older. In short, preschoolers, like older kids, are not immune to psychiatric problems and disorders requiring treatment. Medications serve as one of the options for these youth.

What do we know about the effects these drugs might have on the child years later?

Again, although generally safe over the short term, the older-generation antipsychotic medications have been associated with tardive dyskinesia, an irreversible muscular movement that was noted in some adults who had been exposed to Thorazine-like medications for years; it was later reported in children as well. It is noteworthy that we now rarely use this class of medication in youth. In addition, studies in the field of neurology have shown that certain anticonvulsants may cause gum disease or mildly reduced intellectual development over time.

> **antipsychotic**: A medication used to treat disturbances in the perception of reality (psychosis). Synonymous with *neuroleptic*.
>
> **anticonvulsant**: A medication used to treat seizure (convulsion) disorders. Anticonvulsants are also used in psychiatry for behavioral outbursts and mood swings.

Beyond this, though, we know little about the long-term side effects of most medications, and what we do know is shrouded in myth. For example, many people are concerned about the growth stunting they have read about in children receiving stimulant medications for ADHD despite the fact that this effect has been observed in only a minority of children. Furthermore, our group at Harvard has published a series of studies showing that these are actually growth delays (the children reach their expected height) and are probably related more closely to the ADHD than to the stimulants prescribed to treat it. Unfortunately, few studies of the long-term effects of various agents in children have been available to debunk such myths, due in part to the fact that children have not been taking these medications long enough for their effects to be studied. That is all changing, however, and data from long-term studies should become increasingly available in the future. For example, longer-term (2-year) studies with Adderall XR, Concerta, and Strattera (atomoxetine) show these agents to be effective and well tolerated with no major problems identified for the majority of children and teens who take them.

For now, as a parent who will be responsible for the everyday monitoring of your child while she is on medication, it is important to recognize that some side effects are inevitable because of the way our current medications work in the brain. As I will explain on page 27, we have not yet reached the point where we can isolate a drug's action so that it affects only the targeted function within a brain region or the targeted molecules in certain neurochemicals. This leaves us with medication that can control hallucinations but may also cause muscle spasms and with drugs that alleviate depression but may also sedate the child.

Until we come up with medications that have a very narrow focus of action, parents should be prepared to monitor their children closely for any side effects, short- or long-term, and discuss them with the child's practitioner.

How do the medications work?

We've known for centuries that nerves are the body's messengers and that the brain is essentially an enormously complex network of nerves. Think of the brain as "communications central"—the place where information about what we are experiencing is processed, eliciting certain responses from the body and mind. You want to touch an object, and the nerves in your hand send a message to your brain where other nerves instantaneously set into motion the action of moving your hand to the object. That's a pretty amazing facility by itself. Now add in the brain's capacity to store and analyze information. Over time, these processes produce the overall spiritual and conscious understanding of who you are, what you feel, and your place in relation to others and the world. We call it the human mind, a facility of such mind-boggling sophistication and infinite ability that its workings seem unfathomable.

We still have a long way to go before we unravel the machinery of the human brain, but recent brain research has produced information invaluable to the treatment of psychiatric disorders. Studies of brain structure have shown that some disorders originate in certain regions of the brain, and advances in neurochemistry have revealed that certain brain chemicals may be the source of other problems.

Like other organs, the brain is susceptible to illness. Within behavioral and emotional disorders, these problems are thought, to a large degree, to be related to neurotransmission, or the communication between nerve cells. The medications used in children and adolescents appear to operate by normalizing many of these biochemical disturbances. The scientific community is currently in the process of disentangling which disorder is related to what area of the brain and what neuron-to-neuron pathway.

What happens where in the brain?

The brain has regions that are associated with various cognitive and motor functions. These regions communicate with one another via nerve cells (*neurons*). Much of your emotional processing occurs deep in your brain in the collective region referred to as the *limbic structures*. Disturbances in these areas, such as occur with temporal lobe epilepsy, can lead to rage attacks, deepened emotions, and irritability. Normal inhibitions are thought to originate predominately in the front area of your brain, in the frontal lobe (behind your forehead). Hence, disturbances in inhibition or impulsivity, like those typical of ADHD, appear to have their source located to some degree within the frontal lobes. Another important structure in the brain, called the *striatum,* is related to attention and reward centers. It is thought that problems in this small section of the brain may be important in a wide array of disorders, including ADHD and drug abuse. In addition, certain parts of the striatum are related to your movements. That is why many of the medications used to correct disturbances in reality, such as eliminating hallucinations, may cause muscular spasms or involuntary movements *(dyskinesias).*

> **cognitive functions**: Activities related to the ability to think—take in and process information, reason, memorize, learn, and communicate.
>
> **motor functions**: Activities related to the ability to move.

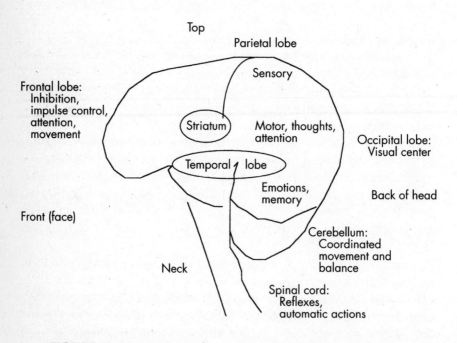

FIGURE 1. Brain areas relevant to neuropsychiatric disorders.

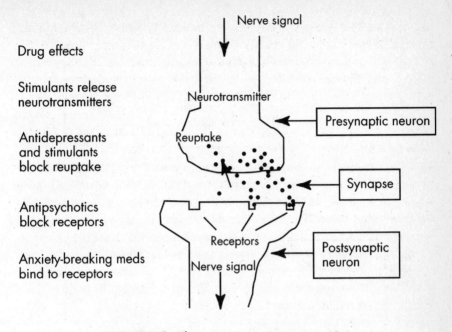

FIGURE 2. The nerve-to-nerve connection.

The brain communicates within itself and with other parts of the body through nerve connections. The area in which the nerve cells connect and communicate with each other is called the *synapse*. Every thought and physical action is related to activity in the synapse. Two or more nerves may communicate in a single synapse, similar to highways merging together. One nerve will send a signal to another nerve cell "downstream."

Nerve communication is carried out by neurotransmitters, such as dopamine, serotonin, norepinephrine, GABA (gamma-aminobutyric acid), and glutamine. Currently, there are thought to be over 200 different neurotransmitters in the brain. Many emotional and behavioral disorders are thought to be related to disturbances in the flow of neurotransmitters from one cell to another.

The synapse is composed of three basic parts: (1) the nerve cell sending the signal (presynaptic neuron); (2) the channel between the nerve cells (cleft); and (3) the nerve cell receiving the signal (postsynaptic neuron). The receiving nerve cell contains receptors, which essentially catch the neurotransmitters, sort of like a complicated baseball glove. Upon catching a very specific area of a neurotransmitter, the receptor will start a complex set of events. Often these events lead to the receiving cell's briefly being "turned on" or "off."

> **receptor:** A chemical structure on the surface of sending and receiving nerve cells that binds or catches the chemical messengers (neurotransmitters), causing other reactions in the nerve cell.

The process of neurotransmission goes something like this: A molecule of a neurotransmitter is released from the sending nerve cell, goes across the channel, binds to the biological "baseball glove," and activates the receiving neuron. The neurotransmitter is then taken back up into the presynaptic neuron by a process called *reuptake.* Reuptake serves two major purposes: (1) to dampen the amount of neurotransmitter in the area between the nerve cells (synaptic cleft); and (2) to conserve neurotransmitter as it is broken down and reused. Not surprisingly, the body is quite an efficient recycling machine!

what happens if reuptake blocked?

Which neurotransmitters are involved in which disorders?

The synapses are the area where the psychotropic medications are thought to act. The psychoactive medications block where the neurotransmitters work (as antipsychotics do) or may act directly to release the neurotransmitters (as the stimulants do) or to block the reuptake of the neurotransmitter (as antidepressants do). Blocking the reuptake allows the neurotransmitter to accumulate in the synapse, making more of it available to stimulate the receiving nerve cell. Prozac, Celexa, Zoloft, Luvox, and Paxil specifically inhibit the reuptake of serotonin and are referred to by physicians as the *selective serotonin reuptake inhibitors* (SSRIs). Similarly, the class of medications called the *tricyclic antidepressants* (desipramine, nortriptyline, and others) acts to prevent the reuptake of norepinephrine and, to a lesser extent, serotonin. Strattera (atomoxetine) blocks only the reuptake of norepinephrine.

Recent imaging and biochemistry studies have assisted us in better understanding what neurotransmitter systems are related to the various neuropsychiatric disorders. It is thought that in some cases of obsessive–compulsive disorder there is inadequate serotonin, which is boosted with the use of selective serotonin reuptake inhibitors (Prozac-like medications). ADHD is thought to be related to deficiencies in the action of both

TABLE 1. Brain Regions and Neurotransmitters Associated with Various Neuropsychiatric Disorders

Disorder	Neurotransmitter	Region
Alcoholism	GABA, glutamine, opioid system	Global, frontal lobes
Anxiety	Norepinephrine, GABA, dopamine	Global
Attention-deficit/ hyperactivity disorder (ADHD)	Dopamine, norepinephrine	Frontal lobe, striatum
Depression	Serotonin, norepinephrine	Frontal lobe, limbic areas
Drug abuse	Dopamine, opioid system, GABA, glutamine	Multiple, hypothalamus, tegmentum
Obsessive–compulsive disorder	Serotonin	Striatum, cingulate
Psychosis	Dopamine, serotonin	Frontal lobe, striatum
Seizure disorders	GABA	Usually parietal, temporal lobes, but generalize to all
Tourette's and tic disorders	Dopamine, serotonin	Basal ganglia, frontal lobe

dopamine and norepinephrine. Not surprisingly, those medications that increase norepinephrine or dopamine appear to be the most effective for the treatment of ADHD.

Unfortunately, the pharmacology is not as simple as it sounds. There is not only a large degree of overlap between the various neurotransmitter systems, but certain neurotransmitters may play a role in a number of different neuropsychiatric disorders. For example, the Valium-like medications (benzodiazepines) affect the neurotransmitter GABA and are used for a wide variety of conditions, including anxiety disorders, alcohol withdrawal, and seizure control.

> **neuropsychiatric:** Related to the interface of
> psychiatry and neurology; referring to the set of mental
> operations that are related to both thinking/emotional
> states and neurological operations.

To complicate pharmacotherapy further, one brain region may be the originating point of a disorder but may also govern other functions. So, when a drug targets that region, it may affect the other functions while it is alleviating the disorder. The striatum, for example, governs movement but also is the source of hallucinations, so when a drug corrects a disturbance in reality, it may also cause muscle spasms. Also, because we have not found a way to isolate the effects of a drug so that only the targeted molecules are affected, a drug may have unwanted effects along with the desired effect. One example is the older antidepressants, many of which, by blocking histamine receptors, not only alleviate depression but also commonly lead to sedation. Fortunately, doctors sometimes take advantage of such side effects, recommending nighttime administration of a sedating drug to a child who has insomnia. Similarly, stimulant medication and some antidepressants (Wellbutrin) used for ADHD may make tics worse, perhaps by nature of their dopamine-enhancing properties. In addition, high doses of agents that affect dopamine may also affect norepinephrine and serotonin.

As a field, we are constantly amassing new information from neuroimaging and other technologies, and we still lack much knowledge about how the brain works—and how dysfunction in the brain takes shape as psychiatric disorders in children (and adults). Although we are narrowing the areas of the brain that are functioning differently in kids affected by different disorders, one of the areas that we do not understand fully is the role of the cerebellum. Previously the cerebellum was thought to be related only to motor coordination, but now we believe it is probably responsible for much more. For example, all of the recent studies looking at brain regions and ADHD have found differences in the cerebellum. Such findings have been reported in adult studies of a host of conditions, including ADHD, schizophrenia, and autism.

Nor do we know much about the cross-talk between the frontal areas of the brain and other regions or the duplicity of neurotransmitters in certain areas (e.g., norepinephrine and dopamine). By *cross-talk*, we mean the communication between the frontal area of the brain, which seems to be where many problems lie, and other parts. We speculate that many of the impulse control conditions, for example, including ADHD, are associated with problems in the front areas of the brain, yet we also know that there are important structures deep in the brain that connect to the front. Therefore we are trying to understand better whether the problems actually lie in the front part of the brain—or whether the problem is located elsewhere, and the problem occurs because the "signal" is not getting to the front. Picture your flight from New York to Los Angeles ending up arriving late. This could have happened because your flight left late, was held up en route, or arrived on time but sat waiting for an open gate. The end result is that you were late. Along the same lines, neurosignals often originate in one area of the brain (e.g., the striatum or occiput) but link to the front of the brain. What we need to know is where the actual problem originates if we are to solve it. We believe it's possible that the problem doesn't lie in the frontal areas alone, because our medications for ADHD that ultimately appear to affect the frontal areas (including the stimulants and Strattera) work directly on brain regions quite a distance from the frontal areas.

If psychological problems are so firmly founded in biology, shouldn't we be able to do a brain scan or a blood test to make sure that my child has the disorder the doctor says he has?

One of the most common complaints leveled against child psychiatry and psychology is the lack of objective methods of testing children and teenagers for what psychiatric problem or disorder they may have. While some biological tests were used in adult psychiatry in the 1970s, virtually no acceptable "biological test," including brain pictures of activity or blood tests, is available yet for the major psychiatric disorders that affect children. Of course, before we get too pessimistic, remember that your child's doctor doesn't use laboratory or other tests to diagnose a common cold or the flu.

If the cause of emotional and behavioral problems lies in the brain, how is it possible that intelligence isn't always affected in children with psychiatric disorders?

Intelligence is a complicated quality, both to describe and to measure. But, you're right—even in the presence of some psychiatric disorders, children score high on IQ tests. ADHD is a notable case in point. Many kids with this disorder have high IQs, and once they are treated so that their symptoms don't get in the way of their concentrating on their schoolwork, they are high academic achievers too. The same is often true of children with anxiety disorders; deficits in intelligence and academic performance are not core problems associated with these illnesses—although the stresses of dealing with the anxiety can certainly get in the way of clear thinking and optimal academic performance.

Why this is so probably has to do with which parts of the brain are affected in the disorder. Work in the field suggests that mood disorders involve the limbic structures of the brain, such as the amygdala and hippocampus (close to the middle of the brain). ADHD involves largely the frontal region of the brain (over the eyes). Other specific neuropsychiatric conditions involve the temporal lobes (near the ears). See the references at the back of the book for more information. There is much that we don't yet know. There is, however, a lot of current interest in the cognitive (thinking) problems that accompany a variety of disorders in kids. These fall largely into the category of executive function deficits. Many of the psychiatric disorders that affect children behaviorally and emotionally also have profound impact on the child's cognitive abilities. We are better appreciating that, beyond improving a child's behavior, we should be carefully evaluating how his brain senses information, processes and packages it, and organizes and carries out various tasks with it. The field is now beginning to treat these problems with remediation, educationally as well as pharmacologically, after the other major problems have been addressed. For instance, it is not uncommon to see a child who has been treated for severe compulsive rituals to be subsequently treated for substantial attentional problems with stimulants or other medicines known to be useful to enhance attention.

Recently there has been a lot more research interest in the executive operations of the brain—the internal "secretary" that is present in most of us but lacking in some of our children with psychiatric disorders. Normally, the brain undertakes many executive operations to assist with planning, execution, follow-through, and the filtering of irrelevant, distracting ideas from relevant, useful ones. Without proper executive function, children often have difficulties with planning simple projects such as preparing themselves for the day, starting a homework assignment, allocating proper time for homework or other projects, and sticking with projects. These youth often space out easily and have severe organizational problems. Researchers such as Russell Barkley and others have theorized that problems with inhibition of ideas and thoughts are fundamental and lead to severe dysfunction in both behaviors and thinking processes in the children and adolescents affected.

> **executive function deficits:** Disturbances in the sequence of mental processes that relate to the ability to plan, initiate, organize, and follow through on an activity. Includes problems with time management, organization, and prioritizing.

If my son's whole problem is neurological, why is the doctor recommending psychotherapy too?

Many mental health practitioners treat psychiatric disorders in children with a combination of medication and psychotherapy, for several reasons. If you read page 19, you know that the current view of childhood psychiatric disorders is that they fit an interactive model. Yes, biology plays a major role in making a child vulnerable to an underlying dysfunction, but exactly which disorders develop, to what degree, and what associated symptoms appear may depend on external factors, including your parenting style, overall family dynamics, and other elements of the child's environment. I have seen many children develop a disorder when their vulnerability to that disturbance due to family history interacted with stress and a learned response to the environment. Perhaps the most telling examples are young people with a family history of depression who become depressed after the loss of a loved relative, friend, or pet. These youth are often already vulnerable to depression, but do not develop the disorder until it is triggered by a life stressor such as a loss. If I downplay environmental factors in this book, it is only because I have seen too many parents mired in guilt over the possible role of the child's home life in causing or worsening the child's disorder. It is not because I believe environment has no import or psychotherapy has no therapeutic value.

Your challenge as a parent is to determine exactly *why* the mental health professional is suggesting psychotherapy for your child. Even today, some practitioners believe children's psychological problems are rooted exclusively in a dysfunctional parent–child relationship that should be resolved via psychotherapy. Other mental health providers are not up to date on the scope of disorders affecting children and adolescents, while still others remain reluctant to recommend medication because of biases or limited knowledge. Asking questions about what might be accomplished in psychotherapy can help you distinguish between a constructive suggestion and an implication that you may be to blame for your child's disorder after all.

A generalized answer to the effect that "psychotherapy is usually necessary in these cases" may be a signal to consider the issue further. A recommendation of psychotherapy (or any other treatment) should be based on the specifics of your child's circumstances, and the doctor should tell you which of those indicates psychotherapy if you ask. Also, because many forms of psychotherapy exist, your child's practitioner should prescribe *specific types* of treatment. Examples include cognitive and interpersonal therapies, behavior modification, family therapy, and many others.

Under the best circumstances, it is difficult to determine whether the family situation is causing, or caused by, an acting-out child and thus how psychotherapy may be of help. Remember, many parents develop specific styles of parenting based in part on the hard-wired personality (temperament) of their child, which in turn may affect that child's development. It is difficult to disentangle whether the child is acting a certain way based on a particular parenting style or whether the parent is reacting to the child's biologically based problem. Autism serves as a perfect example: Mothers of autistic children are not "stone-faced" and generally indifferent to the subtle needs of their children, as was previously believed; let's face it, if your child does not react to your smiles, you eventually will smile at your child less often.

Similarly, the parents of markedly obsessive children will have to change their daily routines to accommodate many of the child's idiosyncrasies. Likewise, parents of irritable children report censoring their discussions and often feeling as if they are "walking on eggshells" to avoid disturbing their children. Mental health professionals sometimes interpret such behavior as a cause rather than an effect of the child's disturbance. If your child's doctor suggests that psychotherapy might prevent behaviors like this from causing or worsening your child's problem rather than saying that psychotherapy can help you determine how much family patterns constitute a cause or an effect of the child's disorder, consider the advice carefully before following it.

A clear-cut case of confusion between cause and effect involved a 14-year-old girl whose severe obsessive–compulsive disorder continued to keep the family awake at night despite 2 years of family therapy. Emily spent every night checking to be sure that doors were not left ajar and that all of the electrical plugs were pulled out of the outlets. The family felt angry, frustrated, and hopeless, and the therapist hypothesized that the family's anger was the cause of the child's acting out. After 1 month of Prozac, however, Emily's compulsive and ritualistic behaviors greatly diminished. Almost immediately, the family reported substantially reduced disruption and chaos, as well as improved relationships between the various family members and Emily. As is the case in many of the children I see, the child's emotional or behavioral state greatly disrupts the family, and appropriate treatment of the problem in the child can often lessen the family disruption.

This is not to say that proactively changing parenting styles via psychotherapy doesn't have a positive impact. Many parents of bipolar and ADHD children I treat feel they are always yelling at their children. They probably are; because of their impulsivity, these children usually have to be corrected often and watched carefully. Even if the child's condition is treated successfully with medication, the parent will need to begin punctuating the positive aspects of the behavior. Children, and also parents, are remarkably responsive to positive feedback, particularly when there has been so little attention to it in the past.

Mental illness can have far-reaching effects on the coping mechanisms of everyone in the family. By the time you seek help for your child's problem, you may have learned some ineffective coping methods, and your child may have underdeveloped social skills. Cognitive therapy with behavior modification can help restore healthy coping mechanisms and reverse some of the impact of living with mental illness for everyone in the family.

In the final analysis, the treatment of your child's problem is multifactorial, just as its cause is. Medication is not an "instant fix" (in fact, most take some time to work), and it is not a panacea. Be open to treatments other than pharmacotherapy, including possibly homeopathic preparations, diet regimes, and anything else that you and the doctor agree has comparatively high benefits for low risks.

My clinical impression is that often medications help reduce the core symptoms of a disorder, thus allowing parents to reset their parenting style to a more positive modality. This combination can propel a child and family to a rapid recovery and ultimately improve family relationships. In countless cases I see, there is a complex interaction between the child's inherent personality or biological constitution and the parenting or family interactions. By identifying the role of your parenting style (and your beliefs about parenting) in your child's emotional and behavioral state, you will be in a much better position to help others understand what might be going on with your child. Be open to the possibility that psychotherapy may be needed to help you reach this understanding.

Also realize that drugs may not be a panacea for all the problems associated with your child's psychiatric disorder. Sometimes a psychiatric disorder forces families to construct a life of limitations around the affected child. While medication may ease depression, control hallucinations, or prevent mood swings, drugs cannot by themselves create a healthy social life for the child or help the child make other adjustments to a more normal life from one founded on disability. This is where psychotherapy comes to the fore.

My child's therapist not only recommends psychotherapy but has stated outright that he disagrees with the use of medication for this disorder, even though the nurse practitioner who referred us to him said it is one option. What should we do?

First, the therapist should have a diagnostic hypothesis of what is wrong and a well-developed plan for intervention. Unfortunately, a minority of counselors continue to work with children and adolescents without a specific understanding of what is wrong. Often, disagreement arises when one of your child's treaters does not have a working diagnosis of what to treat. When there is agreement on the diagnosis, everyone is left with using the most effective known treatment(s) to ameliorate the problem.

When therapy is being tried on its own and is working well, medications may not be necessary. However, if there are persistent symptoms, or no improvement, or an actual worsening in the child's condition during protracted therapy, the therapist should be identifying alternative solutions. If medications have been considered and the therapist voices opposition, ask for an articulation of the therapist's reasons for disagreeing. Try to assess the therapist's knowledge about psychotropic medications, training in this area, and overall perspective regarding nature (biological vulnerabilities) versus nurture (child-rearing practices). Combined psychotherapy and medication treatment is commonly effective for most psychiatric disorders. Thus a medication trial need not raise an either/or dilemma. Moreover, disorders with clear environmental components (posttraumatic stress disorder [PTSD] for one) can respond well to medications also.

In the rare case that you find yourself in the middle of the differing opinions of two providers, you are left to exercise your own judgment, which often includes replacing one of the treaters. I have had children change therapists successfully on more than one occasion when the therapist was against the use of medications or when I felt that suboptimal care was being given. On the other hand, if you have doubts about the evaluation, diagnosis, or treatment recommendations of a prescribing physician, get a second opinion (see page 83) and/or change practitioners.

Finally, be open to the possibility that the psychotherapist might be the least biased source of advice on treatment. Some parents find it useful to speak to a psychologist about considering medication. Since psychologists do not prescribe medication and are experts on testing and psychotherapy, they can often give you an objective picture of the usefulness of psychotherapy and medications in your child's case. Not all psychologists are equally knowledgeable, however. Generally, you will want to consult an experienced, licensed social worker or a doctorate-level mental health practitioner, and don't be afraid to ask whether he or she feels qualified to advise you in this area.

Are there any rough guidelines to when medications are needed and when psychotherapy is preferred so I don't go into this process completely ignorant?

You're wise to try to become informed from the start, because your judgment can be just as important as that of the mental health care providers you consult on your child's behalf. Accept the notion that your child's treater may not know what is wrong: Some cases may be exceedingly complex; some problems are just beginning to emerge with the child's age or puberty; and some treaters have a lack of experience with certain problems. Knowing where each type of treatment is generally preferred can help you spot when a doctor is obviously headed in an unusual direction.

It is prudent to think of using medications for those problems that (1) are known to be responsive to pharmacological intervention and (2) have not responded to nonmedication treatments such as psychotherapy. The order in which medication is used depends on what we know about the effectiveness of the medicine versus other forms of treatment. For example, in children with uncomplicated ADHD, medications are considered the first-line treatment and are viewed as superior to therapy alone. In contrast, medications are not used in adolescents as primary agents for the sole treatment for substance abuse. For depression, most in the field suggest psychotherapy initially or in concert with pharmacotherapy. The verdict is still out on when to use medications for anxiety disorders in juveniles, with most experts recommending a course of cognitive-behavioral treatment before using medications. Children with Tourette's, bipolar, or psychotic disorders generally require medication treatment, with little improvement from psychotherapy alone.

Here are some specific points about particular applications of the two classes of therapy:

- In general, psychotherapies are reasonable considerations as first-line treatment for adjustment disorders and anxiety disorders (but not obsessive–compulsive disorder—very specific cognitive treatments are often used for this disorder, but they are only sometimes fully effective on their own).
- Pharmacotherapy is the preferred treatment in cases of ADHD, Tourette's and tic disorders, bipolar disorder, psychotic disorders, and severe depression. Since mood instability, bipolar disorder, and disturbances in reality often signal serious disorders for which other therapies alone are insufficient, pharmacotherapy should be seriously considered early in treatment of these children.
- Depression is a difficult call. As there is a growing pool of data to suggest its effectiveness, psychotherapy should be considered initially in children with depression, particularly when the symptoms of the disorder appear to be related to a specific stressor such as loss of a friend. On the other hand, specific drugs have been demonstrated under scientific conditions to be effective in reversing the symptoms of depression.
- As discussed on page 41, it's important to understand that psychotherapy often ameliorates other problems or helps kids deal with their disturbance even when it does not change the underlying or core disturbance.

Children who have significant phobias about specific objects, such as animals, that are causing problems might benefit from a form of behavioral modification instead of a minor tranquilizer such as Valium.

Additional information on the hierarchy of treatment choices for specific disorders can be found in each chapter of Part II.

Severity. Mild disorders with few associated problems may require only minimal intervention. For example, children who become nervous in the presence of others may respond very well to a type of focused psychotherapy called *behavioral modification*. Conversely, medications may be considered first when the child's problems are severe or the child is at risk for harming himself or others. Clearly, children who are depressed and suicidal, those who are hallucinating or having difficulty distinguishing reality from fantasy, and those incapacitated by their disorders are potentially good candidates for medication. Less severe cases, such as children with attentional problems who are underachieving despite changes in their routine, also generally benefit from medication treatment.

The Benefit of Combined Therapy. The most common scenario in our clinics is the concurrent use of medications and psychotherapy. Although not well studied formally, feedback from kids, parents, siblings, and schools generally indicates that psychotherapy and medications together have an additive and more lasting effect than either treatment alone. One recent large 2-year study supported this idea, indicating that children with ADHD achieved "wellness" more commonly when treated with medications plus psychotherapy than when they received either treatment alone. Counselors report that children are more attentive to therapeutic issues, pharmacologists report an improved response to medications, and most important, parents notice better overall functioning and quality of life in their children.

Making Decisions Based on the Child's Specific Needs. Given the lack of systematic data guiding treatment, decisions have to be made on a case-by-case basis. After hearing the available therapies (including an array of different types of psychotherapies) described, you should help your child's care provider focus on the *specific* needs of your child. It's far too easy to resort to whatever therapy happens to be readily available rather than to identify and seek out therapies that specifically address what is ailing the child or family. For example, children with obsessive–compulsive disorder should be receiving specialized cognitive-behavioral therapy, not traditional psychotherapy. Traumatized children, on the other hand, may require insight-oriented therapy to process the event intermixed with occasional behavioral interventions targeted at specific symptoms such as panic and dissociation.

Exercise the same curiosity and thoroughness in choosing specific psychotherapies as you would in accepting medication suggestions for your child. If you're not sure you understand why a certain type of therapy is prescribed, ask the practitioner to list your child's specific needs. Do you concur with the list? If not, review these needs with the doctor; don't hesitate to offer parental insight. Once you and the doctor agree on a list of needs, ask the doctor to enumerate the therapies that address each of them before you agree to pursue one or more.

We really trust and like the pediatrician who is urging us to get an evaluation and treatment recommendation for our daughter, and we're worried that we'll end up dealing with new doctors who don't inspire our confidence this way. Can our pediatrician guide us through the whole process?

Assuming he or she has the authority to prescribe medications in general, your child's pediatrician (or family practitioner) is qualified to supervise a psychotropic medication trial for your child. Those who can write prescriptions include medical doctors (MDs)—family practitioners, medical-pediatric specialists, pediatricians, child psychiatrists, and child neurologists—doctors of osteopathy (DOs), nurse practitioners (NPs), and physician assistants (PAs). Other mental health providers who *cannot* prescribe medications include psychologists, who may have a master's degree (MS or MA) or a doctorate (PhD, DSc, DEd, DPhil), social workers (BSW, MSW, LicSW, DSW), and counselors (usually BA or no formal education). Parents often confuse child psychologists—who usually are involved in diagnostic testing and therapy of children but are not qualified to prescribe medications—with child psychiatrists—who are qualified to diagnose, treat, and prescribe medications.

It is important to understand, however, that the authority to write prescriptions is not the only criterion that qualifies a provider to treat a child for psychiatric disorders. For children with serious behavioral and emotional problems, referral to a qualified doctorate-level professional is advised for diagnostics and/or to a child psychiatrist for diagnostic assessment and consideration of medication. A child with uncomplicated ADHD can benefit from good medication management by a pediatrician, family physician, or qualified nurse practitioner. In contrast, a child with depression should be referred to a mental health professional for diagnostic workup and treatment. It would be preferable to have that child see a child psychiatrist (MD or DO) or developmental/behavioral pediatrician for pharmacotherapy consideration; however, if not available, a pediatrician can monitor medications and coordinate care with the mental health provider.

It is impossible to describe a typical health care setting in which you might obtain the care your child needs because there is so much diversity in provider systems and insurance programs such as managed-care programs. Some clinics use a child psychiatrist, who works with the family and child providing both psychotherapy and medications. Other clinics rely on social workers to initially diagnose (triage) a child's problem and work with the family while referring the child to a behavioral pediatrician or child psychiatrist for a medication evaluation. Yet other practices depend solely on nurse practitioners to diagnose and treat a child pharmacologically with referral to a psychotherapist when indicated. In our clinic, families meet with a social worker and have some testing prior to meeting with a child psychiatrist/psychopharmacologist. We refer children to practitioners either in our clinic or to ones geographically situated near the family for specific types of psychotherapy or testing. Ideally, your child would have a prescriber and a psychotherapist working side by side as a team, but that option is seldom available these days. The social worker, psychologist, counselor, or nurse practitioner who can be so helpful to the family system may come from yet another source. In a growing number of medical practices, a psychologist, social worker, or nurse practitioner is in fact the primary mental health professional working conjointly with a prescribing practitioner. In these settings, the psychologist's role varies from providing therapy to being responsible for the diagnosis(es), treatment approach, and monitoring of progress. Given the degree of comfort of the mental health professional, even though he or she cannot prescribe, the psychologist may also serve as a medication consultant with the physician.

Get to know what the role of these various providers is in working with your child's doctor, since they may be the most useful personnel in the office to work with during a trial of psychotropics. For example, many doctor's offices have a nurse working closely with the physician. The nurse is often equipped to talk with you about what to expect in side effects and what constitutes a response to the treatment. Moreover, the nurse will be checking the child's blood pressure and often ordering or performing blood tests depending on the medication. In this scenario, the nurse would be a good contact person if questions or problems arise during the treatment.

For ease in care delivery, whenever possible, try to consolidate your child's care in one setting, particularly if your child has multiple medical and psychiatric problems necessitating multiple treaters and medications. At the very least, try to use providers who have worked together in the past. I work with a number of therapists in the community and generally share their philosophy and overall approach to treating most disorders. When there are differences in perception between caregivers, stay focused on doing what is best for your child.

Everyone except my son believes he should be evaluated for possible treatment with drugs. How do I convince him to be open to this option?

Many kids do not think they have a problem requiring treatment with medications. Some have insight into their problems but don't believe they are serious enough to warrant medication. Some blame teachers, parents, or others for their problems. Others simply don't acknowledge any disturbance in their behavior. Interestingly, children and adolescents with emotional problems such as depression or anxiety seem more open about their problems and more willing to report and receive treatment for them than kids with different psychiatric disorders.

For kids who deny that a problem exists, the best way to encourage acceptance is to initiate frank, nonaccusatory discussions. Be prepared, though, for a battle. In these cases it's difficult for anyone, from parents to teachers to health care practitioners, to get a child to see the light. Be sure to focus on objective facts—the child is failing classes, behaves irritably, worries a lot—rather than subjective perceptions of the problem ("Dad and I are really worried that there's something wrong with you"). Also try to use the words that the child will use in targeting the problem—say you want to help your teenager, for example, with his "problems with teachers" rather than with his "behavioral problems." Always couple the facts with positive comments about the child. These discussions must always acknowledge the child's strengths. Commenting that you know how hard your child has been trying to be good or to do his schoolwork despite the problems will show your undivided support. Likewise, you need to keep reminding your son how much you love him. Say that you want to find out what is wrong and have it treated because of how much you care about him. Remember, even though you may be angry or frustrated by your son's behavior, he is usually feeling even worse about it. Younger children in particular often harbor unspoken fears of being "different" or "not good enough" and consequently losing your love and approval. They need all your patient support to feel safe being honest about their problems with you and the professionals available to help.

An excellent way to convince these children that it's OK to admit to a problem and to get help for it is to offer examples of others who have benefited from treatment. Most kids have had a friend or relative, including a parent, who has been treated for some type of psychiatric or psychological problem. A number of kids I treat for anxiety or panic disorder appreciate knowing that their mom or dad is also taking Xanax, Klonopin, or Zoloft. Although you should exercise discretion in disclosing your own or others' treatments to your kids, by using such examples, you can normalize the disorder(s) and make your child understand that there are others with similar problems. Likewise, by pointing out the other person's positive response to treatment, you can help reduce the hopeless and helpless feeling your child may be experiencing.

Another tack in making your child more aware of his disorder is to describe the problem in terms of a medical condition. However, be careful not to make your child feel as though he suffers from some type of bizarre illness. I tell kids with ADHD that, as in children who wear glasses for poor eyesight, medications will act like glasses for the brain and help to focus their attention. I also stress that having a psychiatric disorder does not mean that a child is dumb and that many of the kids I work with are very smart and hard workers.

Adolescents pose some extra challenges. Distrust of the parent or guardian or doctor is not uncommon among teens who have felt alienated due to their condition. Naturally lack of trust can hinder a teen's compliance and sabotage any treatment. Some older kids fear their parents are just "drugging them" to quiet them down or hold the opinion that Mom and Dad have the real problem and are the ones who need treatment. Kids also may not trust the school and will be reluctant to take medications that need to be registered or administered at school. Some kids, older and younger, simply do not like or trust the doctor treating them and will act out by refusing to take the medication once it is prescribed. Often these children are expressing their own fear this way, and it may help to acknowledge to them that you know everyone involved is having a hard time. Asking specifically what the problem is may help salvage the doctor–child–parent relationship. In rare cases, however, switching doctors may be best. I committed one 5-year-old boy with ADHD and severe oppositionality to a psychiatric hospital, and he subsequently refused to come in and see me or to take any medication I prescribed. After I transferred his care to a colleague, he felt more comfortable voicing (in four-letter words) his opinion of my professional care and is now doing well.

Most adolescents are also reluctant to take medication because they are very worried that it will alter their personality. All you can do is reinforce the notion that medications should not change a teen's personality. If your teen brings up an example of so-and-so who looked like a zombie when on a medication, comment on the lack of information about what was really going on and the individual nature of each case; state firmly that if such a reaction were to occur in your teen, the medication would be discontinued promptly. Medications should help children and adolescents feel better, concentrate longer, feel less angry, or be less hot-tempered, but they should not change anyone's basic personality. You should contact your child's doctor if your child appears sad, agitated, pensive, or anxious, or manifests other emotional states that are out of character while on medication.

Some kids refuse to take medications without giving a specific reason. Since children and teens have an active fantasy life, you would be wise to ask your child what he thinks might happen if he takes medications. You may be surprised by the answer. Julie, a 14-year-old with long-standing depression and anxiety, thought she would have to give up her "skepticism" toward life if she were started on medication. Although she was quite insightful about her depression and the impairment caused by it, such as her having no friends, she felt as though her core image as a cynic would be tarnished if she were on medication. Some kids have been influenced by horror stories from their peers. Tim, a 7-year-old with ADHD, feared that he would get sick if he took medication. It turned out that he had heard of other kids becoming ill on medications at an ADHD support group meeting. Siffon, a 15-year-old girl with trichotillomania (hair pulling) and obsessive–compulsive disorder, was reluctant to take "drugs" because of concerns she had picked up at school about becoming a drug addict.

Sometimes a child's imagination makes him identify negatively with a relative or friend who has a mental illness. Fifteen-year-old Samantha stopped taking the medications prescribed for her depression because she did not want to be like her estranged schizophrenic aunt. Since she knew she was not like her aunt right now, but that her aunt reportedly had tried to commit suicide at one point, she thought that the transition might have occurred as a result of medication. Some kids may not want to be identified with a parent's behavior. Eleven-year-old Todd was so angry at his abusive, alcoholic father that he "wanted nothing to do with" anything his father recommended, including medication that would alleviate Todd's ADHD symptoms and aggressive behavior stemming from oppositional defiant disorder. Thirteen-year-old Eric thought that his Serzone would turn him into a drug addict like his heroin-dependent aunt.

In cases like these, explore the child's thoughts about other family members, the child's problem, and the role of medication. In response, explain that your child is unique and describe how much her circumstances differ from those of any other family member the child is identifying with. To prevent your child from adopting a victim stance, stress the powers she has over her destiny and the need to work with her treatment to get better. Many teenagers respond well to feeling empowered.

My daughter is desperate to get better and wants to know whether medications will cure her. What can I tell her?

The question arises often: Will the medication eliminate the disorder (*be curative*), as in the case of penicillin and strep throat, or will it just reduce the symptoms (*palliate*) while the child is taking the medication, the way insulin reduces blood sugar? This issue is complicated by the understanding that many disorders cycle from mild to moderate/severe disturbance. In other words, many psychiatric disorders will wax and wane spontaneously, totally unrelated to treatment. In these cases, the medications may appear to be treating the disorder when, in fact, the disorder would have dissipated on its own. This is the case with many anxiety disorders, with some cases of severe obsessive–compulsive symptoms, and with mood disorders. After one year of disabling symptoms despite medication and therapy, one 16-year-old girl I treated had a complete remission of her condition (severe depression accompanied by hallucinations) and has done well without any treatment now for 3 years.

---

curative: Eliminating the underlying problem, as antibiotics do when they cure an infection by eliminating the underlying bacteria.

palliative: Alleviating the symptoms but not curing the underlying problem. Narcotics ease the pain of a wound but do not heal the cut.

remission: A reversal of a disorder, leaving no symptoms; the opposite of a *relapse.*

If my child takes medications, will he have to be on them for the rest of his life?

Unfortunately, no one knows how long your child will need a particular medication—or any treatment for that matter. The only way to determine whether someone still needs medication is to discontinue it and see if the symptoms come back (recur or relapse). For the majority of disorders, it's prudent to reevaluate the need for continued medication following a good response of 6–12 months. Rather than stopping the medication abruptly, your doctor may choose to taper it slowly, instructing you to observe your child's behavior closely for deterioration. This strategy is particularly useful in juvenile-onset depression, where medications can be discontinued slowly and restarted upon the emergence of mood symptoms. Tapering medication also reduces the chance of withdrawal symptoms caused by the sudden removal of certain compounds. Choose when to taper medication carefully, however. It would not be wise to try it, for example, during school when it is important that your child perform well if he is finally doing well because of that very medication.

> **relapse:** The recurrence or worsening of a disease or disorder; the opposite of *remission*.
>
> **withdrawal:** Mental, emotional, or physical reactions to quick discontinuation of a medication.

Aren't the medications addictive?

There is a big difference between addiction and dependence. Children are not *addicted* to the medication since they do not get high (euphoric) on the medication or alter their behaviors to find additional tablets of the agent to "feed" their habit. *Dependence* means the child finds she does not want to stop the medication for fear that her symptoms will return. It's important to understand that dependence may occur and is not necessarily bad. Children and their parents are dependent on a number of people and things around them. Individuals with vision problems rely on their glasses, adults driving to work on their cars, and carpenters on their tools. All of us are dependent on friends and family members. In this vein, most individuals receiving medications develop a trust that the medication is effective and safe and will help eliminate distressing psychiatric symptoms.

A poignant example of typical and reasonable dependency is Abigail, a 15-year-old girl who successfully battled substance abuse but still suffered from depression. Treatment with Effexor at 75 mg twice a day improved Abigail's mood, peer and family relationships, and school performance, and she told me she was very concerned that I would stop her medications now that she was feeling better. She did not want to "go back to feeling like #!&*" but was worried about her need for the medication. After 1 year of being symptom-free, she has done very well after having the Effexor tapered off slowly.

I have seen many cases of youths with obsessive–compulsive, Tou-rette's, and anxiety disorders who have similar concerns. Although I know of no reference to describe this phenomenon, I have observed that kids or their parents often know intrinsically when medications can be tapered, and it is at these times when kids lose their need for the medication. Concerns about reliance on medication are common and can be dealt with easily by sharing them with your child's doctor.

The more serious problem is addiction, a concern voiced most often in families whose children are receiving controlled substances such as stimulants (Ritalin, Dexedrine, Concerta, Adderall) and those with Valium-like properties (Klonopin, Ativan, and similar drugs, called benzo-diazepines). Although there is potential for abuse with these medications, the overall risk that a child will develop an addiction to his own medication is very small. Isolated cases of kids "popping," "sniffing," or taking extreme amounts of their medications to get high have been reported—including one case of a child breaking up Ritalin tablets and then sniffing them—in our clinic and elsewhere. Your careful management of your child's medication coupled with your ongoing observation of your child will help prevent this problem or help you identify it quickly if it emerges.

> **controlled substances:** Classes of compounds categorized by the U.S. Drug Enforcement Administration as potentially addictive.

Won't taking these drugs lead to later drug abuse?

Many parents fear that taking psychotropic medications now will predispose their child to taking street drugs later. These concerns are amplified when the child's prescription is for a controlled medication such as Ritalin, Metadate, Concerta, Dexedrine, or Adderall (which are stimulant-type agents) or the Valium-like medications. To date, no long-term data or case series (a number of individual cases) support this concern. In fact, a recent study that evaluated the world's literature on this topic found that treating kids with ADHD using stimulants *reduced* the risk for later substance abuse by half.

When such kids do develop a later addiction to a street drug, it is usually the underlying disorder and the environment in which they are involved that place them at risk for later addiction. Young people with depression, anxiety, or ADHD and conduct disorder, for example, are at risk for later substance abuse largely by nature of their conduct disorder. One 16-year-old boy who has been on Strattera for 5 years found that the medication was relatively effective in treating his ADHD but that many delinquent behaviors related to his conduct disorder failed to respond to a multitude of interventions. Recently he admitted to daily marijuana use as well as occasional LSD use. The boy's parents suspected that his stimulant medication had resulted in later drug abuse, but I believe his underlying conduct disorder was more likely a pathway to drug abuse.

> **amphetamines**: Drugs in the stimulant family with chemical structures resembling naturally occurring compounds such as epinephrine; used to treat ADHD, narcolepsy, and depression.

Another common pathway to substance abuse is living in an environment of tolerance for illicit drug use, as in schools where daily marijuana smoking is not considered aberrant. Parents who are using or abusing illegal substances also put their children at risk by nature of genetics and poor modeling. This contrasts with parents taking prescribed and licit medications, which serves as a good model for their children.

Finally, consider the possibility that not being treated for the disorder—optimally or at all—may lead your child to future drug abuse, as was the case in one study of ADHD children growing up. The demoralization, distressing symptoms, and underachievement that often result from leaving a psychiatric or psychological disturbance untreated are known to place children at risk for later substance abuse. Think of this risk as reminiscent of the well-known medical risk of stroke following untreated hypertension. Although the hypertension may not be life-threatening, poor blood pressure control may show up as serious complications decades later. Similarly, your child's disorder may not seem very severe today, but leaving it untreated can subject your child to an accumulation of harmful secondary effects that may very well put the child at risk for adolescent substance abuse.

Won't these drugs just mask the underlying problem?

This concern is perfectly logical. We all know it would make no sense to do nothing but give Tylenol to a child with a persistent fever. Therefore, it's natural to worry that psychotropic medications may harm the child by ignoring the disease while treating only the symptoms. Unfortunately, we know little about the underlying biological "core" disturbance associated with most disorders, so we have little recourse for treating it directly. In general, we see medications as being extremely useful in lessening the severity of disabling and distressing psychiatric symptoms—no mean feat when you consider how debilitating those symptoms can be when not treated. Let's assume, though, that we could treat the core disorder. Would that free the child from all harmful effects of having had the disorder in the first place? Often it would not. To use a medical example, even when an earlier conflict has been processed properly, residual effects from the disorder typically remain. A fat-laden diet may predispose you to develop blocked arteries in your heart. Although you may correct your diet as soon as you learn about this risk, the need for treatment could remain if your arteries are already clogged.

> **core disorder:** The primary or major problem.

Most parents who ask me this question really mean "Aren't these disorders caused by some unresolved conflict that requires psychotherapy?" Since we know that certain disorders are inherited and associated with brain changes seen in brain scans, I tell them, it is unlikely that the underlying disturbance in these cases can be addressed solely with one of the talking therapies. When children have emotional or behavioral difficulties that are related in part to earlier environmental problems, or when severe trauma or other stressors have primed the child to have specific symptoms, psychotherapy may indeed be helpful, but often after the child's symptoms are treated with medication. In some cases, until the symptoms are ameliorated, the child cannot effectively engage in therapy. When an obvious stressor is identified—at school, for instance, this could be a learning problem or victimization by other kids—medications are not the first-line treatment. Instead, elimination of the stressor from the environment would be tried first. In the case of other persistent or unsolvable problems, that might mean switching schools, which might or might not be practical. If you are concerned that your child's practitioner is ignoring the existence of some such stressor or some underlying conflict, ask whether there are psychotherapy options available. In many cases, both medication and psychotherapy are advisable.

What happens if we opt not to accept medication treatment
for our child?

As discussed earlier, among the many factors to consider is the specific
disorder and its severity of effect in the child's life. Complicating your decision about using medications to treat your child is the possible risk involved in leaving the disorder undertreated if other interventions have
been ineffective. It's not difficult to imagine the day-to-day demoralization
and helplessness heaped on a child with an unremitting disorder. If you
think back to your own childhood, you will undoubtedly remember the
majority of negative events you endured. In simple terms, bad things have
a way of sticking with us. This fact is confirmed by adults who express
sadness over the years during which they believe they were unnecessarily unhappy while their anxiety remained undiagnosed and untreated during their adolescence. Coupled with this emotional angst is the very real
underachievement that children experience when they have an untreated
disability. Debilitating failures, socially, academically, and otherwise, can
begin in childhood and dog the boy or girl into adulthood. Children with
ADHD, for example, are often vocal about the frustration and poor self-
esteem they feel over consistently getting poor grades in school. Children
with bipolar disorder may be at risk for suicidality or harm to others if not
treated. Children with psychosis may have worsening of their brain functioning if left untreated. Logically, then, it is probably not in your child's
best interest to ignore a disorder that is causing observable impairment.
In making this important decision, you may want to ask yourself whether
you owe it to your child to try a medication that could actually help—after
all, it would not be recommended unless indicated for your child's problem.

Unfortunately, the vast majority of studies showing medication effectiveness are short-term ones (6–8 weeks long), so we are left speculating
that there is a quality-of-life improvement in children as they mature
when their psychiatric disorders are treated appropriately. We do know
that studies in children with depression indicate a higher rate of suicide in
those untreated, leading experts to speculate that treatment of the disorder may reduce the ultimate risk of a tragic outcome. We also have en-
couraging data for ADHD, the disorder on which the greatest amount of
long-term data has been gathered. One recent study in children with
ADHD suggests that Ritalin improves multiple aspects of the child's well-
being after 2 years of follow-up. Another multiyear, government-funded

study of the long-term effectiveness of various types of treatment for ADHD indicates the essential role of medications in long-term management of ADHD. Finally, a study done in New York showed that children with ADHD assessed in adulthood who had been treated with stimulant medications had fewer crime and drug-related problems than a similar group of untreated children with ADHD.

Parents should not be greatly discouraged by the lack of firm evidence on other disorders. Medicine has been plagued by a similar dilemma over the long-term implications of treatment for years. Despite 20 years of intensively managing blood sugars, for example, only recently has the long-term beneficial effect of close sugar control on reducing diabetes damage in grown-up children been highlighted. Similarly, studies showing the long-term positive effects of consistent blood pressure and cholesterol control in reducing cardiovascular problems are relatively recent. In both cases, though, physicians considered the short-term benefits sufficient to justify treatment. In a similar way, the fields of developmental pediatrics and mental health ascribe to the notion that the treatment of psychiatric disorders will reduce the risk for later problems related directly (such as suicide in the case of depression) or indirectly (such as substance abuse) to the initial difficulties.

Aren't drugs really expensive?

Yes, they are. Why this is so is another question, and there is no short answer. I certainly cannot defend some of the high costs of medications; however, many of the prices appear to be related to tangible expenses incurred by the pharmaceutical industry. The industry explains that the pricing of medication is based on research and development, manufacturing, regulatory, legal, and distribution costs, as well as pharmacy markup and profit margin. It is helpful to realize that drug development is lengthy and expensive. A standard patent for the pharmaceutical industry is 17 years. On average, it takes 3–5 years to study a medication in the laboratory and then another 4–5 years to test in humans. It costs approximately $100–200 million to bring a drug through the process to the market. At a regular development pace, the pharmaceutical company has about 5–10 years to sell the drug without cheaper generic competition. Therefore, in the relatively short period of time available, the pharmaceutical companies need to recover their costs of development and marketing while making a profit from the medication. This, of course, doesn't make it any easier on your pocketbook. One thing that can ease the bite is to watch for more competition. Ask your pharmacist to be sure to let you know when new, less expensive brands come on the market.

How can we possibly handle the cost of all this medication without prescription coverage in our insurance plan?

Fortunately, many current insurance plans do offer coverage for prescriptions. In fact, I instruct parents of the children I treat to select plans that will cover the prescriptions, even if the plans exclude me from their provider network. The costs of medication can range from $20 to $400 monthly. If prescriptions from your child's mental health practitioner are not honored for copayment, consider asking your child's primary-care provider to rewrite the prescription. Most providers will consider this option if provided with the medical records and/or a letter indicating the current diagnosis and treatment by the specialist. If you are paying for the prescriptions, it is important to note that prices vary among pharmacies, buying in bulk (100 instead of 30 tablets or capsules) will reduce prices, and using larger pill sizes (such as one 100-mg tablet split in half instead of two 50-mg tablets) will be less costly. To avoid wasting money on unused medication, consider filling only part of the prescription when initiating treatment in case your child has an adverse reaction and must discontinue that agent. Better yet, ask your child's doctor if samples of the agent are available. Also, ask your insurance company if 3-month supplies are available by mail. Often the 3-month plan allows for refills of noncontrolled medications, significantly reducing the copay. Finally, some generic medications may substitute for the more expensive brand name agents. If the cost of the medication is prohibitive, or if you find yourself financially prohibited from purchasing medications, some of the pharmaceutical companies have limited free access to their products. Either you or someone in your prescriber's office can contact the maker of the prescribed medication for more information. Generally, these services are time-limited and need to be renewed frequently. Or get the Patient Assistance Directory from the Pharmaceutical Research and Manufacturers of America (202-835-3450 or *www.phrma.org*). Another source of medication may be the local, state, or federal government's assistance programs for children (Medicaid or the Children's Health Insurance Program [CHIP]). These programs often allow limited medical/psychiatric and prescription coverage for children and adolescents.

CHAPTER 2

THE PSYCHOPHARMACOLOGICAL EVALUATION
Finding Out What's Wrong

Surgeons do not operate without having a good idea of what is wrong with their patients, and mental health professionals should not prescribe medication or other treatment until they have a handle on your child's psychiatric or psychological problems either. The only way to obtain a reliable diagnostic assessment is through a thorough professional evaluation of the child and, in most cases, the family as well.

A psychopharmacological evaluation can have many parts, depending on the needs of the individual child. You may already have completed some parts of the process, or you might just be setting out after a consultation with your child's pediatrician. Perhaps you have already received a referral to a mental health professional from the pediatrician or your child's school. The sequence in which your child is evaluated for diagnosis and pharmacological treatment and the types of practitioners you consult will depend in part on where you live and what types of mental health facilities are available locally and through your insurance plan. You may not need all the information in this section, but I've attempted to answer all the questions that parents most frequently ask me and my colleagues. These run the gamut from "How do we find the best doctor for an evaluation?" and "What does an evaluation involve?" to "How can we prepare our child for the evaluation?" and "What kind of conclusion should we expect?"

In this day and age, of course, the question of cost almost always arises, and it is a good idea to know what you can expect. A solid 1- to 2-

hour assessment by a physician—the basic evaluation—should cost an average of $200–600 today. However, additional psychological testing may cost up to $800, and neuropsychological testing may cost $1,200–2,500 or so. If you are advised to pursue this extra testing, be sure to contact your insurance company for information on coverage.

As parents, you are in a position to supply much of the information that an evaluation will take into account, so it is crucial that you diligently report on your child's current symptoms and history, as requested. It's also important to have realistic expectations of treatment and to be familiar with the risks and benefits of any medication(s) ultimately recommended for your child. Because you will be dealing with specialists, the evaluation is a good place to start gathering expert information. Think of the evaluation as the beginning of your active collaboration with your child's mental health practitioners.

Our pediatrician gave us the name of a child psychologist and a child psychiatrist to consult about our son's apparent depression. We don't want to waste time but don't know how to make the choice. Which one should we call?

If your son's depression doesn't appear severe, there's a good chance that psychotherapy will be the treatment choice, so you might want to try the psychologist. If the evaluation inspires your trust in this practitioner, you may want this person to take charge of your child's subsequent treatment. If the depression is severe, there's a chance that medication will be advised, in which case you'll need an authorized prescriber anyway. As discussed on page 42, many doctorate-level child psychologists are the best choice for an initial diagnostic workup, but if drugs seem inevitable, you might want to get a psychiatrist involved from the start.

Obviously part of your decision will have to be determined by practicalities such as who is included in your managed-care insurance program. Other issues to factor in include the office or clinic's proximity and the availability of related services should referrals be needed. The referring pediatrician should be able to advise you of the latter.

After my 12-year-old daughter suddenly started talking about voices she hears, we rushed her off to the pediatrician, who examined her and said nothing seemed wrong except possibly stress and suggested we could see a psychologist if we wanted to. Should we?

You should definitely get an evaluation of your daughter's problem right away, but I suggest you ask for a referral to a child psychiatrist instead. Disturbances in reality and mood swings generally indicate a serious problem that is probably going to require, at the very least, a medication consultation. If your pediatrician does not know one, other sources of reliable referrals could be the American Academy of Child and Adolescent Psychiatry in Washington, DC (see "Resources"). Without going into any detail about your reason for the request, you might also consider asking the school's guidance counselor or psychologist if a list of mental health professionals is available from the school.

Our daughter has had various behavioral and emotional problems over the years, and she has seen her school psychologist regularly. Now, though, the school is recommending a professional evaluation, and I have no idea what it involves. What is it likely to include?

The school's recommendation is likely an acknowledgment that whatever has been done for your daughter in the past is no longer helping her. As in any field of medicine, the first step in treating a disorder or disease is to figure out what is wrong. Your daughter's school is urging you to do just that, and until you're confident that you have a reasonable idea of the nature of the problem, you should not proceed with medications or any other treatment.

As to what will be involved in your daughter's evaluation, quite frankly, there is no cookbook method. The diagnostic process, or workup, differs greatly from clinic to clinic but should feel more like an ongoing process because information turned up in one step will determine the next step. The common thread in all psychiatric evaluations is the attempt to figure out what is wrong with the child. Because all children are embedded in their environment, the diagnostic workup must look at the impact the environment has on the child, how the child's problem is interfering with the environment (as in disrupting the family's home life), and how the child's problem and environment are interacting (as in school performance).

A psychopharmacological evaluation will be dedicated largely to diagnosis, just as any psychiatric evaluation will be, but you and the evaluator will also want to be sure your child has no major medical or neurological problems and that medication, if considered, can be taken safely because, for example, the child has no cardiac problems or seizures. The basic exam generally will be a 1- to 2-hour meeting with a medical practitioner who has mental health expertise or experience (such as a developmental and behavioral pediatrician with extra interest and experience in the care of these children, or a child psychiatrist). This exam should include a discussion with you, the parents, as well as an interview with and/or observation of your child, often in your presence. During this discussion, the practitioner should review relevant information from previous treatments or concerns forwarded by your child's school.

The table on page 60 shows other possible parts of an evaluation. Your child may undergo more thorough diagnostic testing, including structured psychiatric interviews, which are careful, nonbiased assessments of all possible psychiatric conditions that may affect your child and are often available only in academic or tertiary referral centers. Rating checklists may be completed by you or your child's school, including the Conners Rating Scales, Brown ADD Scales, and Child Behavior Checklists. The practitioner may also suggest cognitive testing, including the Weschler Intelligence and Achievement Scales. Often social service representatives work in concert with medical practitioners to assess family dynamics (interactions that may be causing or exacerbating your child's behavior) and to investigate any concerns about abuse or neglect of the child.

Your child won't necessarily participate in all of these during the initial workup. Depending on the child's situation, in fact, you may tap these resources as needed over months or even years. As children develop, new problems or symptoms may emerge, calling for new or repeated testing. Children who are not doing as well academically as their intelligence level indicates they should, for example, may undergo repeat tests to determine whether there is quantifiable evidence of change in their condition.

Again, each clinic is different, but let me walk you through a typical experience at our clinic. After initial contact with our clinic, parents are asked to complete a questionnaire covering many aspects of their child, such as current problems, school issues, legal involvement, past treatments, and the like. The parents then meet with our social workers (not in the presence of the child) for 1 hour to discuss the family's concerns, interactions with the child, and to provide parental support (or referral to a family therapist if necessary).

As a next step, the child and a parent go through testing, including a structured psychiatric interview administered by a trained clinical assistant (or psychologist in some centers) to one of the parents (and to children over the age of 12). This interview covers all symptoms of all possible psychiatric disorders, with the goal of generating a list of psychiatric problems that should be considered. The child will undergo an abbreviated form of cognitive testing to get an initial simplified assessment of the child's learning disorders, general intelligence, and areas of weakness or underachievement. Then the parent and child meet for 1 hour with the medical practitioner, who now has the information gathered so far and the child's past records at hand. On average, a workup at our clinic takes about 2 months to complete. If, in the process, other concerns arise, such as the possibility of a medical problem like seizures, the child is referred to the appropriate physician for follow-up to assist in diagnosis. Similarly, should we conclude that psychotherapy should be the first line of treatment tried and that psychopharmacology will be considered if psychotherapy is not effective or if the child's condition deteriorates, we refer the child to a therapist who can help.

As to your situation, your daughter's school may very well have referred you to one or more professionals who can evaluate her. Be sure to ask the practitioner you call what you should expect from the evaluation.

What's the very least we should expect from an evaluation?

The *basic* psychopharmacology assessment involves a practitioner's taking a careful history of the child, family, and environment in a 1- to 2-hour session. Common to all evaluations is this face-to-face interview in which

---

WHEN TO SEEK HELP

Seek a professional evaluation when your child exhibits any of the following symptoms:

- Self-harm or suicidality
- Threats of dangerous harm to others
- Severe outbursts or anger attacks
- Auditory or visual hallucinations (hearing or seeing things that are not there)
- Marked withdrawal or isolation
- Weight loss with no medical cause
- Severe substance abuse
- Bingeing and/or purging (vomiting) food

TABLE 2. Elements of the Psychopharmacology Evaluation Process*

Test	Reason
Family evaluation (with a social worker)	To determine what family dynamics, if any, may be contributing to the child's problem; suggest having a family behavioral modification therapist involved in case
Psychosocial and school assessment (teacher or guidance counselor contact)	To assess child's peer functioning; determine academic and behavioral performance at school
Psychological testing (with a psychologist)	A broad group of tests that assess the child's emotional and cognitive (thinking) functioning; suggested if there are learning problems not attributable to psychiatric disorder
Neuropsychological testing (with a psychologist)	Extensive and specific tests to evaluate a child's thinking or information-processing abilities
Structured interviews (varied)	Detailed questions about your child's history; available only at certain clinics
Medical assessment (pediatrician)	Physical examination and laboratory studies; suggested prior to using medications and when there are concerns of a medical contribution to the disorder
Medication evaluation (medical personnel)	Thorough history of the child and his or her current and past emotional and behavioral problems; review of above

*This table represents potential assessments for children with behavioral and emotional disorders. The evaluation process varies greatly, depending on the region of the country, the type of practice, and the circumstances of the child.

the health care provider elicits a thorough description of the current problems and symptoms as well as information on any previous treatments your child has undergone for this problem.

A family and developmental history of the child is essential. Your family's record of either diagnosed or suspected psychiatric or substance abuse problems will provide your doctor with valuable clues as to what may be wrong. For example, it is not uncommon to see Tourette's disorder in children of parents with obsessive–compulsive traits and vice versa. Likewise, sons of alcoholic fathers are at increased risk for a number of problems, including alcoholism, ADHD, and conduct disorder. Children of parents with anxiety, depression, or manic–depressive illness are at higher risk to develop those disorders.

A thorough developmental history of your child from birth to the present can reveal several types of useful information. For example, you can pinpoint exactly when various symptoms began, which can help you determine whether they are developmentally normal events or signs of an emerging disorder. You can also spot the existence of certain pervasive developmental disorders such as autism and the occurrence of types of separation anxiety.

What should we look for in a doctor to perform the evaluation and possibly to treat our child as well?

You have the right to know about the person to whom you are entrusting your child's diagnosis and care. Don't be afraid to ask a prospective health care provider about his or her credentials or experience, and be wary of one who gets irritated by your questions. More commonly, though, the doctor will be only too happy to tell you about his or her qualifications. These are questions you can ask to get a synopsis of the professional's philosophy, training, and experience:

- "How many children like my son [or daughter] have you treated before?"
- "What modalities do you commonly employ in your treatment plan?" Evangelical or closed-minded responses should raise a red flag. Remember, medical practice is based on science and not philosophy or immutable beliefs.
- If the doctor is at an academic center, "What is your subspecialty or area of specialization?"
- "What is your training [degree and medical and postgraduate residencies]?"
- For psychiatrists, "Are you board certified in child psychiatry?"
- "Are you affiliated with an inpatient unit to which you refer patients when necessary?"
- "What is your background in internal medicine, neurology, or pediatrics?"
- "How many years have you been in practice?"

Be aware that some states, such as the Commonwealth of Massachusetts where I practice, allow patients access to their doctor's license status, any complaints lodged with the state medical board, and any medical malpractice cases filed against a physician. If you want this information, contact your state's medical board or Division of Consumer Affairs.

Perhaps the most anxiety-provoking moments in the psychopharmacological treatment of your child are the initial visits to the doctor for an evaluation. During this period, you will be dealing with such crucial issues as the diagnosis and the prognosis. You will also be involved in making decisions about what medication your child will be taking. Since you are ethically and legally responsible for your child, you will be authorizing and choosing what medication is to be used. If this alone doesn't drive you to the need for Valium yourself, you will also be the "maestro" of medication monitoring and the one who coaxes (or bribes) your child to go to the clinic for routine checks. Given this responsibility, you will need close and frequent contact with the physician's office to effectively adjust your child's medication. It is preferable to find a practitioner who can monitor your child's progress after doing the evaluation. So, in choosing an evaluator, consider whether this person is available to follow your child, and, if so, whether you want to deal with this professional on a regular basis.

> **diagnosis**: What is problematic with the child.
>
> **prognosis**: What is expected to happen to the disorder and the child over time.

Our pediatrician's group now includes several nurse practitioners, and when we inquired about having our child evaluated for behavioral problems, we were advised to see one of them. Are these professionals as qualified to perform an evaluation as our usual pediatrician would be?

Nurse practitioners have completed a master's degree in nursing *and* have additional intensive clinical training in specific areas of expertise. Nurse practitioners typically work in concert with a physician, often being supervised by the physician on more complicated cases. Generally nurse practitioners can prescribe all classes of medication, though that varies somewhat by region. Nurse practitioners have taken an increasingly important role and are increasingly relied on to diagnose and treat a host of psychiatric disorders in children and adolescents. As is the case with phy sicians, there are good and not-so-good practitioners, so you should feel free to talk with a referred nurse practitioner to get a good idea as to his or her training and experience in working with children.

The receptionist at one doctor's office gave me a long list of information that I would have to bring to the evaluation from my child's school. Can't we keep the school out of it for now, to protect my child's privacy?

The child's current academic functioning and peer relationships are two major domains in a child's life that fill out the child's history and current status. The school (or day care center for younger children) is in a unique position to provide input in these areas, so the doctor should have this information from the start if dependable conclusions are to be reached. You are right, however, to want to protect your child's privacy. Doctors are required to treat patient information with strict confidentiality, and schools are expected to keep diagnostic and treatment information confidential, but they don't always do so. I require parents' signatures to release any information about their child to the school, but because you cannot be sure who will see your child's school file, I discourage parents from providing the school with the child's entire evaluation. The school does not need to see information gathered during an evaluation that is not relevant to the school's direct needs. Instead, have the treating physician write a succinct letter with the major diagnosis and reason for the communication (such as special education needs or medication administration).

The recent proliferation of privacy-related laws has restricted the flow of information between schools and parents to begin with. In many states school faculty and staff are not allowed to advise parents that their child seems to have problems that would warrant a mental health evaluation; nor are they permitted to report on their observations of how a child is doing during a medication trial. Obviously this means that your child's privacy may be better protected than it was in the past, but it also means that collaboration between parents and schools in the interest of a child's improved mental health can be restricted significantly. On the other hand, you should have no problem as long as you authorize contact between school and practitioner for continuity-of-care needs. To make sure you understand the law's potential effect on your children, read about the law at *www.hhs.gov/ocr/hipaa*.

As to what an evaluator will require from the child's school, just be sure to get a specific list when you call to make the appointment.

Failure in either the social or the academic domain can be devastating to a child's self-esteem and adult future, which is why most schools are diligent in reporting to parents any academic or behavioral disturbances observed in the school setting. Many children, in fact, are initially referred for evaluation by the school. In academics as well as peer relationships, knowing when difficulties arose in the classroom may be a tip-off to the diagnosis. For instance, children with long-standing academic difficulties may suffer from ADHD. Conversely, the abrupt onset of academic decline may signal trauma (posttraumatic stress), an adjustment reaction (persistent reaction to a stressor), severe depression, substance abuse, or bipolar disorder. Difficulties in specific classes may flag either a child–teacher conflict or a learning disability (such as reading).

You too can provide perspective on the child's social world, but your child spends most of his day at school, and that's usually his largest arena for social interaction with both peers and adults. By giving input regarding your child's peer relationships, the school provides additional clues about what may be wrong.

Solid relationships with an acceptable peer group are a positive sign in any child, while the inability to make meaningful attachments with others is a common feature of autism or pervasive developmental disorder. Autistic kids may play with other children but not interact directly with them. For example, 8-year-old Joey, who is autistic, will play cars while other kids play with cars, but he will not interact with the other kids directly or crash into or honk at the other children's cars. Depressed children may withdraw or isolate themselves, and anxious kids may be inhibited in meeting new peers. The school can state not only what the child's relationships look like now but whether they have changed. A child who has been interactive in the past but is now withdrawn may be suffering from depression, whereas one who has never really connected with peers (or family) may be autistic.

Will I have to get the information from the school, or will the doctor contact the school directly?

As a parent you can be very helpful in providing an inventory of your child's school performance by retrieving meaningful information from the school or day care center and bringing this to the practitioner's attention. Similarly, school-based testing and recent progress reports are informative. Forms for filling out information on the child's behavior and academic performance can also be sent to the school; the practitioner will supply them and then use this data to arrive at a "score" for various factors. Two widely used behavioral scales that provide a mechanism for a teacher's input are the teacher report forms of the Child Behavior Checklist (for a wide variety of behavioral and emotional problems) and the Conners Rating Scale (for ADHD). Each practitioner handles this part of the evaluation differently. To save time, ask what might be needed from you when you call for an appointment.

Will my child be directly involved in the entire evaluation?

Caregivers differ in the constellation of family members they talk with during the process. Sometime during the evaluation, the parents (or guardians) and child should be spoken with about the problems as well as the options for treatment. Although direct interview with the child is important, the literature shows that the parents' report, particularly in children under age 12, can be a more accurate account of the emotional and behavioral problems of the child. In my practice, I commonly hear children report that "everything is going great" only to find out they are failing four classes and have three detentions weekly.

As to other involvement, obviously if psychological, cognitive, neuropsychological, or other tests are called for, the child will participate. Never hesitate to ask the doctor what to expect from these testing processes.

How should I prepare my child for the evaluation?

Preparation for your child depends greatly on the child's attitude toward being evaluated in the first place. Children and adolescents vary widely in their reaction to the news that their parents are going to take them in for a mental health evaluation. If your child expresses opposition, remember that you have made the decision to pursue an evaluation for good reasons, and I suggest telling your child that the decision is nonnegotiable. The most important thing is to get the child in for the evaluation.

When you discuss your decision with your child, be honest (using explanations appropriate for the child's age) about why you think an evaluation is necessary. Don't hesitate to bring up the problems that you and the child have been experiencing, but try to avoid negative comments or blame. Say, for example, "I know it bothers you that you've been having trouble with your friends" rather than "You're causing so much trouble in the neighborhood that I don't have any choice."

Your child's willingness to be evaluated may depend on the type of problem the child has. Youngsters with mood, anxiety, obsessive, and psychotic symptoms are often easier to get into a practitioner's office because they can more easily connect the distress in their lives with some type of thinking problem. Those with more externalizing disorders, such as oppositional defiant disorder, may tend to deny their problem or blame it on others and thus are more likely to resist the evaluation.

The child's reaction may also depend on her age. In general young children tend to be more malleable, but they may also be governed by typical fears of doctors. If you know your child is afraid of "shots," for example, assure her ahead of time that she will be seeing a "talking doctor" who does not give shots.

Adolescents can be more difficult and may even try to sabotage your efforts by oversleeping or not coming home from school on time for the appointment. Again, frank discussion of the child's problems may help, but the evaluation is so important to your child that this is a situation where you can feel justified in resorting to bribery if reason fails. Of course, you don't have to word your offer as a bribe. Tell your child that you have chosen this doctor very carefully and are confident that the evaluation will not be too unpleasant but that you know the child will not view it as fun and therefore you would like to reward the child afterward. Offer to take the child to a movie or make a stop at the toy store, depending on the child's age and interests. With adolescents, the disorder may dictate the child's level of cooperation too. Teenagers with anxiety or sadness tend to be easier to get into an evaluation; those with oppositionality or irritability are usually more difficult to engage in the process.

Whatever the child's age, be prepared for the child to be closed-mouthed once you're in the practitioner's office. Teenagers especially, but really all children, usually aren't thrilled at the prospect of talking about their problems with a stranger. It may help if you assure your child (again, especially teens) that whatever is said in the doctor's office will be kept confidential. But don't be too concerned if little Billy refuses to talk to the doctor at all. Considerable information is gleaned simply from observing the child. Also, the evaluator will be taking much more than firsthand impressions of your child into account in making conclusions. All practitioners are aware that children often act differently in their office than at home, school, or with peers, so they do not rely solely on what they see or hear face to face.

Beyond actually getting your child to the evaluation, the best thing you can do to help your child through the process is to make sure you understand and are comfortable with what will be happening along the way. Children and parents both come to this point in their lives with trepidation. Sometimes these fears and doubts coincide, and sometimes they are different, but you cannot very well assuage your child's fears until you've eased your own with reassuring knowledge.

Both parents and children have understandably adverse reactions to certain tests or questions when they haven't been apprised of their purpose. If you don't understand exactly how the results of a test or your answers to a line of questioning will contribute to an accurate diagnosis and ultimately benefit your child, stop the proceedings, ask, and don't move on until you do understand. I've seen many parents and children become offended by certain questions about the child's mental and emotional state when I have failed to state beforehand that I need to cover all bases and that I know not all questions will apply to all patients. I have also seen children become very agitated during tests such as computed tomography (CT) scans and magnetic resonance imaging (MRIs). These tests are noninvasive, but they make some children (and adults!) feel claustrophobic.

Will the evaluation include a physical exam?

Whether your child's evaluation includes a physical exam depends on whether your child has had a complete checkup by the pediatrician that includes all the elements required for psychiatric diagnosis and psychopharmacological evaluation. Generally, children who are being considered for medications should have a thorough medical check, including a physical examination, by their pediatrician to ensure that (1) the child is well, (2) an underlying medical problem (such as low thyroid hormone) is not causing or exacerbating the child's psychiatric disorder, and (3) the child has no major medical problems (such as heart defects) complicating the use of medications.

All medical conditions need to be brought to the attention of the mental health practitioner who is evaluating your child. In particular, a clear history of neurological or other conditions that are closely related to psychiatric disturbances should be made available. Additionally, any previous or current medical problem that may put your child at risk with certain medications should be brought to the attention of the doctor. These could include not only heart ailments but also bone marrow problems or liver disease.

What is the purpose of the "psychological testing" that the evaluator has recommended?

The evaluator may refer your child to another psychologist for additional tests for two reasons: (1) learning disabilities not caused by a psychiatric disorder are suspected and/or (2) the evaluator cannot reach a diagnosis based on the information gathered so far. Specific learning problems like reading or math disabilities can be picked up by specific cognitive testing. Personality problems, problems with distinguishing reality, and certain types of anxiety can be unmasked during particular types of testing referred to as *projectives*. The projectives include the famous inkblots (Rorschach) and other tests that help determine what may be wrong with your child.

Currently psychological testing costs an average of about $500 and includes tests of your child's thinking processes and intelligence (cognition) as well as Rorschach and other interpretive (projective) tests of how your child views himself and his interaction with the environment and others.

If there's something wrong with my child's brain, won't she have to have some kind of neurological tests?

Not necessarily. We now know that ADHD, for example, is caused by a disturbance in the brain, but the presence of specific symptoms sometimes elicited by behavior rating scales is generally all that is needed to diagnose this disorder. In contrast, it is not uncommon to complete the full barrage of tests, including blood tests (see page 181), in a child who develops prominent hallucinations.

If your doctor is concerned about certain types of seizures, he or she may order an electroencephalogram (EEG). This painless procedure may require your child (and you, the brave parent) to stay awake most of the night so that she will sleep during part of the EEG since abnormal brain wave activity is often brought out during phases of sleep.

EEG: Electroencephalogram, used to measure electrical activity in the brain.

Your doctor may also be concerned about possible problems with the way the brain was formed (congenital abnormalities) or may want to be sure there is no ongoing change in the brain substance. Although these conditions are thankfully infrequent in children and adolescents, brain pictures are useful in identifying aberrant blood vessels (arteriovenous malformation), growths (tumors), and damaged areas (infarcts).

Two major types of scans are used to take pictures of the brain: a CT and an MRI (also referred to as NMR, or nuclear magnetic resonance). Both scans are safe for children and adolescents. Although the scans are painless, many children feel claustrophobic in the scanning equipment or are bothered by the "knocking noises" and become quite anxious and agitated. More than one of my patients has had a panic attack in the scanner. Talk with your child about the machine and what it is doing, and also inform the scanner technicians as to how your child is feeling or may react (such as punching the technician). Mild tranquilizers from antihistamines (such as diphenhydramine) to stronger agents such as Valium-like medications or other sedatives (chloral hydrate) may be necessary to keep your child from moving excessively during the procedure.

CT scan: Computed tomography, a detailed, cross-sectional picture of structures in the body and brain made by using X-rays.

MRI: Magnetic resonance imaging, a nonradiating imaging technique that produces better resolution (sharper images) and more varied pictures of structures of the body and brain than CT scans (see preceding definition).

What's the purpose of the blood tests the doctor ordered?

Whether blood tests are considered necessary depends on a number of factors in your child's case. In general, they should be done only to gain specific information that will help the doctor figure out what may be wrong with your child. It is important that you understand their purpose so that you can assure your child that they are justified—especially with a child who fears needles and whom you've assured would not get any "shots" from this doctor. Ask the doctor for an understandable explanation and for help in preparing your child if necessary.

Children with behavioral difficulties, for example, may be asked to have a ceruloplasmin or lead level test. Whereas lead exposure and elevated levels may cause behavioral and intellectual disturbances, elevated ceruloplasmin levels indicate a treatable metabolic disorder called *Wilson's disease*. Both high and low thyroid hormone levels may cause or worsen underlying behavioral or emotional problems in children. Similarly, genetic testing may unveil less common problems such as fragile X (resulting in mental retardation), and metabolic testing may unveil metabolic diseases that may have mental health ramifications. However, despite our field's attempts and parents' wishes, *no blood testing is available to diagnose any of the psychiatric disorders we treat in children and adolescents.*

How do we know if the amount of testing recommended is excessive?

As with any medical test, it is important to have a notion that each test ordered is going to help in understanding what is wrong or in treating the condition. Tests should not be ordered simply for liability protection, academic interest, research without consent, or compensation to the institution or practitioner. For example, more specific neuropsychological testing, which may cost up to $1,200–2,500, should be reserved for cases of complicated learning disabilities or learning difficulties not adequately addressed in more basic psychological testing. Likewise, lab tests should be done for sensible reasons. For example, some clinics suggest expensive "biochemical analyses" of children's brain or blood. These tests, which run up to $1,500, have yet to be validated scientifically and do not provide a foundation for treatment. Again, your best protection against unnecessary tests is to ask the purpose of each and every one.

Beware of practitioners who recommend lots of expensive tests but spend little time on the interview. Neuropsychological testing does not replace a thorough history taken by the doctor in determining psychiatric disorders.

The doctor keeps referring to my child's problem as a "disorder" and referring to something called the DSM. Our pediatrician never used these terms—what do they mean?

A disorder is a constellation of symptoms or problems that have unifying factors such as what caused it (*etiology*), what is wrong (*pathophysiology*), what happens over time (*course, prognosis*), and what treats it. The doctor's main, but not sole, concern in the evaluation is to identify the *core disorder,* which comprises the major symptoms or elements of the disorder. For example, a child with ADHD may display some behaviors such as a temper, but the core disturbances in ADHD are inattention/distractibility, impulsivity, and hyperactivity. Since children often have aftereffects (*sequelae*) to their disturbances, it can be helpful to disentangle what is a core feature of the disorder and what occurs secondary to the disorder. Children with depression (core symptoms of sadness, irritability, low energy) may develop a lack of confidence, which is not a "core" symptom.

DSM stands for *Diagnostic and Statistical Manual of Mental Disorders,* a book published by the American Psychiatric Association that contains a standardized method of diagnosing major mental illness across the life span. The *DSM* (now in its fourth edition, *DSM-IV-TR* [2000]) entails two major aspects of scientific study: validity (are these really disorders?) and reliability (do different practitioners seeing the same patient make the same diagnosis?). The *DSM* has been a great asset to psychiatry by legitimizing the empirical studies behind it. This is crucial since no psychiatric diagnoses can be made on the basis of laboratory or imaging tests alone. Furthermore, it gives credence to emerging information on new treatments because the *DSM* has defined exactly what constitutes a specific disorder. Clinicians reading a study on a successful new therapy for schizophrenia, for example, can be confident that what the researchers called schizophrenia in their study is the same thing that the clinicians see and call schizophrenia in their practice.

In the evaluation interview, the doctor asked many questions that scared me, such as whether my son ever felt suicidal. Won't these questions just put dangerous ideas in his head?

Asking about sensitive mental health concerns such as suicidality does not place the idea in your child's head. In fact, young people are frequently relieved to be able to talk openly in a safe environment about these often internalized feelings. (As I said on page 66, it is often the children with more externalized problems such as conduct disorders who are less open to discussing their problems.) Sixteen-year-old Sean, for example, was brought in for an evaluation because his pediatrician thought that his low energy might have been related to depression. In addition to many depressive symptoms that he had not discussed with anyone, Sean indicated that he had been suicidal for almost 3 months but had felt ashamed to tell his parents and "scared" of the feelings. The interview proved to be a catalyst not only for the parents and son growing closer but also for open communication by the parents about his depression and better assessment of his response to treatment by them.

> **intervention**: Action taken to treat a child's disorder.

Fifteen-year-old Susan reported to me in front of her parents that she had copied the key to the gun cabinet and was planning to shoot herself the following week. I have seen parents stunned by their children's responses to questions, reports spanning from feeling depressed or anxious to having obsessions or hallucinations. So please remember that discussion that may very well cause anxiety in you is having the opposite effect on your child and may in fact save the child's life.

The mental status examination during which such direct questioning occurs is considered the physical examination of mental health and is a crucial part of the basic interview. It is a standard part of all psychopharmacology evaluations. Generally it involves questions asked directly of your child to find out how the child is feeling and to assess the child's thinking abilities and process. The doctor may ask the child if he is bothered by something in particular, if he is sad or mad, and if he is hearing voices or seeing objects that others are not. The questions may be directed to you as well. Sometimes your child may be asked to do simple calculations or recite a series of numbers backward. Do not be offended by the type of questions covered; again, many questions may not apply to your child.

The mental status examination may also include a subjective appraisal that the provider makes during the evaluation. While the evaluator is observing your child and interviewing both of you, he or she may be mentally answering a running list of questions such as these: How is the patient dressed? What is his pattern of speech? What is his sense of reality? Is he suffering from any memory lapses? Is he attentive to the examiner? Does he appear anxious or depressed? How does he relate with the parent(s) or the examiner? Although the mental status examination is a good time to explore various aspects of how your child thinks or feels, don't be alarmed if your child doesn't respond openly or isn't "sick" when evaluated. A competent child psychiatry practitioner will realize that children may not appear disturbed during an interview.

We haven't had a final report from the doctor yet, and I'm worried that he's going to tell us nothing is wrong because Jenny acted perfectly normal in his office!

Many parents become alarmed when their children don't manifest the particular symptoms of concern during the actual meeting with the practitioner. Remember, the symptoms of the disorder occur as interactions between the environment and the child. Some problems, such as academic difficulties, may appear only at school. The practitioner evaluating your child is no more likely to base his or her conclusions only on your child's behavior in the office than a cardiologist would discount the chest pains you report having while walking upstairs simply because you don't have those pains in his or her office! Children may not be inattentive or hyperactive in the structure of a practitioner's office; however, given the school and home environment, they may have fulminant and disabling ADHD. Likewise, depressed children may "hold it together" during the examination, only to fall apart at home. Traumatized children may have the bulk of their difficulties at night, and psychotic kids may not be hallucinating in the presence of their practitioner. In contrast, some children will act worse at the evaluation. I commonly see children who are irritable and angry because they had to see the doctor or because, for example, they were refused a soda prior to the evaluation.

We've put our child through all of this testing, and now the doctor says she's not sure what's wrong. Why is it so difficult to diagnose my child's problem?

The goal of the evaluation process is, of course, to come up with a diagnostic hypothesis of your child's problem. However, the fact that certain disorders may be just emerging and that more than one disorder may be present at one time (see page 20) sometimes makes it difficult to nail down a specific diagnosis. If your doctor expresses doubt, ask for an explanation of exactly what is confusing him or her. Remember, too, that you can be invaluable in observing other symptoms that may have been missed or may arise with time or a change in the environment.

In many children, for example, mood disorders, bipolar disorder in particular, may be difficult to diagnose. Whereas depressed adults can usually verbalize being "down" and often exhibit a characteristic sadness, depressed children often can't express their feelings clearly and may display confusing symptoms such as anger or temper tantrums rather than sadness. All of your insights and powers of observation may be called into play in making an accurate diagnosis if your child has a mood disorder.

I currently treat a 12-year-old boy who had a family history of depression and who was brought in because he was somewhat anxious, isolating himself, and sometimes appeared sad to his parents. He "thought" something was awry but was unable to be more specific and denied frank depressive symptoms or feeling down. We opted to follow him, and his parents observed him diligently. Over the ensuing 4 months, he withdrew further from his family and friends, had difficulties in school, and noted feeling sad. In follow-up visits it was more apparent that he was suffering from depression, and he was started in psychotherapy.

This is a typical example of the collaborative process that accurate diagnosis often requires: I explain my concerns and speculations to the child's parents and ask for their help in watching for certain symptoms. Sometimes the power of suggestion leads parents to amplify the symptoms of the disorder, but I have found that it is much better in the end to identify a possible symptom than to overlook it. If you fear that you're reading something into your child's behavior that doesn't exist, discuss what you've observed with the doctor, who should be able to help highlight meaningful observations. Also, you'll find that you will get quite proficient at distinguishing the significant from the transient, developmentally appropriate behavior of your child—just as you learned to tell the difference between typical fussiness and real illness when your child was an infant.

Unraveling children's psychiatric and psychological disorders poses many challenges to even the most astute diagnostician, not the least of which is finding the fine line on the continuum between normality and abnormality. Some symptoms of diagnosable psychiatric disorders overlap with the signs of a typical reaction to a stressful event. It's perfectly natural and normal, for example, for a child to become depressed or anxious following the death of a loved one. But if the child's depression or anxiety is protracted, the child may be suffering clinical depression that has been triggered by the stressful event. Or if the child begins to have excessive fears of losing a parent every day, a separation anxiety disorder may be at work. Here again, your ability to observe the child over time is invaluable to the diagnostic process. You may be the only person who can inform the doctor of how long, how consistently, and how intensely the child's symptoms have been appearing. The doctor, on the other hand, will be in a position to make distinctions between mental illness and certain medical illnesses—such as hypothyroidism (low thyroid levels)—that mimic the symptoms of mental illness. The doctor should also, through a diligent evaluation, be able to uncover the possibility of any trauma (such as sexual abuse) that could be causing symptoms that look like mental illness.

Yet another challenge stems from factoring in age and developmental level. Simply put, what is normal behavior for a 2-year-old could be signs of a disorder in an 8-year-old. Take excessive activity in a preschooler. Lots of activity may be totally normal, but the absolute inability to stop, the severity of the overactivity, or other co-occurring problems such as aggression toward other children may signal a problem. Many children are active in prekindergarten; however, a very small group of excessively active children are unable to tolerate the structure and "down time" required of them in nursery school and "flunk out." These excessively active children may have ADHD—or they may simply need another year to "grow up" before they are ready for nursery school. Sometimes only time will tell.

We have already discussed the fact that children's psychiatric disorders usually stem from a combination of biology and environment (see pages 10–13). The challenge for the diagnostician lies in knowing how much weight to give each factor in evaluating the child for disorders. Examples of how depression may arise when an environmental trigger brings out a biological predisposition have been given in earlier sections (pages 19 and 20). In other conditions, such as autism and pervasive developmental disorders, the genetics appear to be more powerful than the environment. Clearly, there are a number of cases in which the environment has tremendous impact on later problems. A multitude of sometimes severe and impairing psychiatric symptoms may arise in children who have been severely neglected or abused, and temporary symptoms may show up in a child who has just had a single traumatic experience. But in every case, the effect of the environment needs to be balanced against the level and impairment of the child's response.

Many children are subjected to environmental stressors such as parental separation, but only a minority of children develop persistent and disabling symptoms. It is up to the evaluator to determine whether a child's symptoms are the transient (temporary) products of a single traumatic experience, small or large, or a more permanent (or recurring) result of hard-wired temperament or impairment. Complicating matters is a third possibility: a more permanent result of a very severe, repeated trauma, such as ongoing neglect or abuse. So, a large part of determining what is wrong and whether it qualifies as a psychiatric disorder is deciding how much of the cause is biological (genetic), how much environmental, and how much the interaction between them.

Children with mood disorders are a good example of hard-wired response to an environmental stressor. These kids will cry or become irritable at the drop of a hat and with only minor provocation: We call this *mood reactivity,* an exaggerated response to an event. Some of these children over-respond to limits placed them, like 6-year-old Irma, who throws a tantrum when asked to put her toys away or to go to sleep.

Differentiating inherent from external causes in a child's problems is even more difficult when major stressors exist within the family. For example, financial problems and parental separation, unfortunately common problems, often result in a certain type of response from the child, who is trying to adjust to the situation. When does that typical and expected reaction become a problem? It depends on the severity of the child's reaction, how long the symptoms last, and how seriously impaired the child becomes. Studies show that the vast majority of kids whose parents have separated or divorced have some type of reaction, such as sadness, anxiety, or more overt acting-out behavior such as oppositionality or rebelliousness. Usually this behavior is self-limited, and the parents and siblings can deal effectively with it by talking and maintaining a nurturing home environment. Yet a smaller group of these children may have prolonged, severe difficulties such as extreme reluctance to leave the remaining parent or caregiver, leading to a child's refusal to go to school or play with his friends. These children might benefit from individual or group therapy to discuss the parental separation and what it means to them, as well as more specific treatment for their anxiety if it persists.

In such cases, the children are experiencing substantial anxiety that is impairing their ability to function and can be traced to a very specific event within the family. Unfortunately, in many other cases, far too much emphasis is placed on the immediate cause, or trigger, of the child's problems. Although there are clear cases in which a stressor appears to be the major cause of a child's behavior (such as severe trauma), the event may not be directly related to the disorder. Many parents wonder, for example, if a fall out of a high chair caused their child to develop ADHD. It often emerges, however, that the child was overactive, perhaps resulting in a fall in the first place. Since we have no method of truly assessing what leads to what, it is useful to keep in mind that there is an important interaction between the environment and your child's biological constitution.

As parents, you can, in fact, play a great role in helping the evaluator understand the distinct role of each in your child's problem. I have seen several children whose parents have claimed the death of a pet was the sole cause of their child's continued sadness (*dysphoria*) when, in fact, a 6-month depression is much more likely to result from an underlying vulnerability (such as *mood reactivity*) to depression that was merely triggered by the event. Using your common sense and knowledge of what seems to be an appropriate response to a situation will help you tease out what is normal versus what may be an overreaction to a situation.

> **mood reactivity**: An excessive response to a typical environmental stimulus or stressor, such as a child's extreme anger at normal parental requests.

This is why time is such an unavoidable element in diagnosis. By identifying continued *patterns* of reactivity to typical stressors, you can be very helpful in identifying an underlying vulnerability for a psychiatric disorder. *Persistent* exaggerated responses to an event can be a tip-off to a problem. Children who have *repeated* severe temper tantrums after a typical parental limit is imposed, such as on TV watching, may be oppositional or have a mood disorder.

In these cases, the hard-wired traits of the child interact with the environment to produce the explosiveness. Unless you and the practitioner understand that both factors are involved in causing the problem, the child's behavior is very easy to misinterpret and thus impossible to resolve. Outsiders might naturally think, for instance, that a child who defies parents' commands to turn off the TV simply has a discipline problem rather than a diagnosis like oppositional defiant disorder. A child who refuses to go to school may be misunderstood as "lazy" or "stupid" if her parents don't understand how powerful the interplay of inherent anxiety and the trigger of school is in their child. Returning her to school without recognizing the problem may make her more anxious and more adamant about not going to school. A child who gets very anxious 2 months before an assigned oral book report may not be just "overreacting" but showing the signs of a social phobia.

Understanding the conditions under which a child's disturbances occur is essential to coming up with an appropriate treatment plan. When, for example, I evaluate a child who is excessively anxious about or during school, I assess the school placement and home situation, and if I cannot find any apparent reason for the anxiety, I suggest behavioral modification. Medication intervention is then considered if there are severe symptoms or for those times in the year that are predictably problematic such as the beginning of the school year. These simple and effective treatments often substantially lessen the impact of the child's anxiety, reduce family conflict, and greatly improve the child's social and emotional state. But as you can see, getting to the root of the problem to come up with this treatment can be a long haul.

CHAPTER 3

THE DIAGNOSIS
AND TREATMENT PLAN
Laying Out a Strategy to Help Your Child

Now that the evaluation is completed, you should have a diagnostic hypothesis from the evaluator, along with an initial treatment recommendation. The phase you and your child are entering may be the most difficult in the diagnosis and treatment process. Now you must deal with the full reality of your child's problem and its possible treatment, and many parents find that all their lingering doubts and fears come to the surface. "Is the doctor's diagnosis correct?" and "Does the proposed treatment seem reasonable?" are questions that every parent asks—and *should ask*. Don't allow your child to be treated until you are satisfied that the practitioner's explanation of what is wrong fits your child's picture.

Once you believe you and the practitioner are on the right track toward helping your child, the nitty-gritty of medication trials becomes important. Exactly how do you know that the drug being considered is safe for your particular child? How will the proper dosage be determined? How will your child's school be involved in the treatment? Medication trials require patience and diligence from everyone involved. Knowing as much as possible about what to expect will help you and your child hang in there while the optimal treatment is formulated.

The doctor gave us a diagnosis following the evaluation,
but my wife and I have doubts. Should we agree to the treatment
the doctor suggests?

You should agree to treatment only if you are satisfied that the practitioner understands your child and your concerns and has accurately assessed
the problems. If you are not in agreement with the diagnosis, explain the
reasons for your doubts; in so doing, you might reveal something you
overlooked before that will warrant reconsideration. Also ask the doctor
to explain all the reasons for believing your child has this disorder; you
may learn something that will put you in agreement after all. At the very
least, you may learn more about what symptoms you should be looking for
and can agree to return to discuss the treatment at a later date, after careful observation of your child.

When I saw 10-year-old Sue, who had been getting anxious every
morning before school, the only conclusion I could reach was that she
might have separation anxiety. The girl seemed very shy and essentially
refused to talk during the interview, so she revealed almost nothing about
what she was experiencing. Her parents were no more satisfied with my
tentative conclusion than I was, so we agreed that they should go home
and observe their daughter carefully for the symptoms of separation anxiety that I laid out for them. I also asked them to question Sue closely
about her feelings. It did not take long for Sue's parents to determine what
had been going on: Sue had been experiencing motion sickness on her
long bus ride to school. Once this was discovered, I prescribed Drama-
mine, which alleviated the motion sickness and almost immediately resolved her anxiety.

Sue's was an unusually simple case, and yet it illustrates how easy it
can be to misinterpret a child's behavior. Your child may have far more
complex symptoms that defy a straightforward diagnosis. The point is that
if either you or the doctor has doubts about the hypothesis resulting from
the evaluation, you should keep searching for answers. If you remain dissatisfied and the doctor refuses to budge, seek another opinion (see page
83).

If you're simply feeling reluctant to use medications for your children, do some independent research into the disorder and the treatments
considered effective for it (in addition to reading the appropriate chapters
in Parts II and III of this book). You should be able to get reliable current
information from the American Academy of Pediatrics or the American
Academy of Child and Adolescent Psychiatry (by phone or the Internet;

see "Resources"). Also contact support groups to talk to parents who have been through the same ordeal. You can locate support groups by asking your mental health professional for a list, by calling 800 information, by calling the American Academy of Child and Adolescent Psychiatry or the National Alliance for the Mentally Ill (see "Resources"), or by considering the list in the "Resources" section of this book. What you learn may affirm the doctor's recommendation, point to alternatives you can discuss with the doctor, or help you formulate the questions that will elicit the information you need from the practitioner.

One more source of abundant information is, of course, the Internet. Many authorities will, justifiably, warn you to be cautious about what you read on the Web. You undoubtedly already know that just plugging the name of a disorder into a search engine will produce a long list of websites, some of which may be sponsored by radical self-interest groups or other dubious sources of reliable information, and it's not always easy to sort the wheat from the chaff. But I urge you not to let the need to be discriminating keep you from tapping this rich resource. Most major disorders that affect children (autism, anxiety/panic, obsessive–compulsive disorder, tic/Tourette's disorder, bipolar and mood disorders, ADHD, learning disabilities, substance abuse) have very organized, highly articulate parent support groups that have established very sophisticated, user-friendly websites. These websites often link to articles, chat rooms, general information, referral sources, or professional organizations with more facts and advice. The chat rooms serve as a major disseminator of information and also serve to support parents (especially busy parents who simply cannot make it to support group meetings). Many parents I know have made discoveries on the Web that might not have revealed themselves in any other way.

For example, a parent of a child with autism spectrum disorder related to me that he believed (rightfully) after reading about these disorders on the Web that he has always had a variant of Asperger syndrome. He reported that it was very useful both to himself and to his child to realize this. Many parents note that they have discovered they have or had conditions similar to those their children suffer from: most commonly ADHD, anxiety disorders, motor tics, and depression.

Naturally you should beware of any website whose main purpose (or even a significant goal) is to sell you anything. With that caveat in mind, you should know that the pharmaceutical industry has stepped up to the plate and developed excellent websites with updates, links, and other resources related to their medications (especially those with FDA approval in children). Such websites are generally accurate, are updated frequently, and link to major parent support groups and the National Institutes of Health's related information. Always balance proprietary (corporate) information with unbiased independent sources, but don't deny yourself the help you can get from these websites.

The important thing is that you make no move until you feel comfortable doing so. Leaving your child untreated *for a short period* is unlikely to have any harmful effect. In many cases, a child's parents and I have opted to wait a few months prior to starting medications. Although in my experience I rarely see remissions, I have seen a few cases in which the symptoms of depressive and anxiety disorder lessened and the child never required medication treatment. The parents of a 12-year-old girl who was going through menses and had a history of 4 months of moderate depression, despite counseling and no obvious stressors, opted to continue her in counseling and to use pharmacotherapy only if her symptoms continued or worsened. She spontaneously improved 2 months later and was doing well at 2-year follow-up. In this case, her parents and I kept tabs on her symptoms with a clear plan delineating when to intervene with medications.

So, don't rush the process. If you have serious doubts about using medications, wait and carefully observe the symptoms of your child's disorder over time. Maintain contact with the treating practitioners about your plan. If your child gets better, then your hesitancy in initiating medication treatment was well founded. If your child continues to have problems, or they worsen, you now have more data on which to make your decision. Either way, if you are carefully watching your child, you win. You may never "like" placing your child on medicine, but should you decide to take that route, you will have the satisfaction of knowing you've weighed all the pros and cons and engaged in informed decision making.

Parents are often reluctant to accept a diagnosis if they feel the evaluation process was inadequate or rushed, if previously relevant information was not reviewed, if the essentials of the case were not captured, if the diagnosis given does not seem to fit their child, if the diagnosis is divergent from their initial thoughts, and when the parents are in denial of any problems in their child. I comment to parents after discussing my diagnostic impression of their child's case that it is important that they feel my explanation fits with what they have been observing in their child. In other words, parents have to have confidence that what the evaluator is describing as the "core" features of the disorder applies to the child being seen.

In some cases, I will tell parents that their children have traits of a disorder or that I am concerned that a disorder is currently emerging (such as severe depression or schizophrenia) but that not enough of the symptoms have surfaced for me to give a concrete or confident answer about what is wrong. In those cases, I tell the parents what I am looking for and ask *them* to follow up to provide me with more information. In that way, the parent becomes my eyes and ears and is more involved in the process, as well as being more confident in the diagnosis when it is established.

When should we consider getting a second opinion?

Second opinions serve the purpose of having your child reevaluated from a different perspective as well as either reaffirming your confidence in the first diagnosis or legitimizing your concerns about it. That does not mean, however, that everyone should seek one. If you are satisfied that your child's doctor has a solid understanding of what is wrong and the treatment, don't feel obligated to seek an alternative opinion.

In today's medicine, most practitioners welcome the opinions of others. In that vein, requesting another opinion, particularly about a child who is not responding to treatment or whose case has been difficult, is best served by direct talk with your child's doctor. It certainly helps all involved in the process to be frank, polite, and respectful to the initial doctor. If you wish to continue with that practitioner, I suggest being supportive of the care he or she has been providing and sensitive to what the practitioner would like from an outside evaluation.

Also, since you will probably be seeking out a highly specialized doctor for the second opinion, you will have to endure the usual waiting time to be seen; remember, if the second doctor has a full patient load, this doctor may not be available to follow your child through treatment.

Finally, you have to be prepared for the decisions a second opinion might force: Once you have the information you were seeking, how will you integrate it with any current treatment plan? Both providers may arrive at the same diagnosis but take different clinical approaches and use different judgment in establishing a treatment plan. Neither may, in fact, be "wrong." In that case you may have to make a subjective judgment on which provider to go with if neither agrees to a compromise plan. Are you prepared to switch providers if necessary?

If you get a completely different diagnosis the second time around, you may have to seek a third opinion to confirm one or the other. Therefore, before seeking another opinion, be sure you know what is moving you to seek it, the basic diagnosis or the prognosis and treatment recommendation. Don't expect miracle cures or major breakthroughs from a second doctor, and do a little soul searching to make sure you're not just looking for reassurance that in fact nothing is wrong with your child at all. Consider the process a success if you gain useful insight into your child's condition or if you are reassured that the current diagnosis and treatment recommendation are correct.

To save time, can we just ask another doctor to review the information gathered in the first evaluation and give us a conclusion?

It may be tempting to try to save time and money this way, but to get an objective second opinion, you will need a reassessment of the clinical situation and previous treatments. Although in our group practice we curbside one another frequently for a quick alternative opinion, the information passed on is whatever the primary practitioner perceives. That means if the primary physician has the facts incorrect or has some bias that the second doctor doesn't know about, it will be difficult to spot an error based on the data provided. One thing you're after with a second opinion is anything the original evaluator has missed, so it is much more fruitful to start close to the beginning.

Won't our current doctor be offended—and uncooperative—if we seek another opinion?

You have the right to request a second opinion without the blessing, or even knowledge, of your child's doctor. *As a parent, you need to do what is in the best interest of your child.* If possible, it is generally advisable to discuss your wish for a second opinion with the original evaluator, who may be able to give you the names of some doctors who can help with the case and hence see it as a collaborative event. Most physicians, particularly those who are sharing your frustration with repeated nonresponse to various medications, welcome outside consultation. Indicating that you are appreciative of this doctor's input to date and that this information will help to complement the ongoing treatment plan facilitates this discussion.

How do we find the best possible practitioner to give us a second opinion?

Generally, a second opinion should come from a doctor with a more specific knowledge base than the first one had. For children who are thought to have behavioral or emotional problems necessitating medication, referral to a child psychiatrist, pediatric psychopharmacologist (who is a child psychiatrist specializing in diagnosis and medical management), developmental pediatrician, or pediatric neurologist is suggested. Although generally not familiar with the details of using medication, a child psychologist may be very helpful in diagnostic and systems consultation. Either your child's practitioner or managed care/HMO provider can suggest another physician, or you can speak to other parents through the nationally linked support groups for most of the neuropsychiatric/psychiatric disorders affecting children.

The doctor admits he's not sure what is wrong but says Ritalin has proven helpful in improving hyperactivity like the behavior our son shows. Should we try it?

I strongly suggest having a firm diagnostic hypothesis before treating. It sounds as if your doctor may have accurately put a name to one of your child's *symptoms* but has not fully identified the *syndrome* and therefore has not yet named the *disorder*. It is crucial to distinguish among these three terms in any evaluation, diagnosis, and treatment recommendation. While certain drugs do seem to have a specific effect on a particular symptom, the practitioner should always be treating the entire constellation of symptoms that makes up the disorder—and, as I've said, in many cases, more than one disorder. To blindly prescribe medication in the hope that something will prove to be a panacea for all that ails the child is irresponsible. It will also be ineffective in pinning down a diagnosis. The fact that the medication doesn't work will not eliminate the possibility of a specific disorder. Remember, surgeons carefully assess individuals to figure out what is wrong prior to operating. And you don't blindly administer cough suppressant medication without considering *why* someone is coughing: pneumonia, common cold, or asthma?

Sometimes, however, it may be difficult to pin down an exact diagnosis because a child may have many, but not all, of the symptoms of a particular diagnosis. In these cases, the most likely diagnosis may be followed by the initials *NOS*, which stands for "not otherwise specified." Examples exist for all childhood disorders. For example, bipolar disorder NOS indicates that most of the criteria for bipolar disorder are present and that these symptoms are causing significant daily problems in the child's life ("functional impairment"). Thus, the provider may recommend interventions used to treat actual bipolar disorder.

> **syndrome:** A group of related symptoms and other objective findings. Posttraumatic stress syndrome, for example, is a group of symptoms that have been observed in people who have suffered a significant trauma.

Should I be concerned about the doctor's recommendation that we try medication first, rather than something less invasive?

Much depends on weighing risks versus benefits in your child's individual case. Sometimes, especially when the disorder is serious, it is appropriate to try medication right away, along with other types of treatment, as long as there is a good chance the medication will work and is not too dangerous. I know you've been exercising parental vigilance to keep anything unknown from passing your child's lips, but for certain disorders, such as bipolar disorder and schizophrenia, pharmacotherapy is the accepted first-line treatment. If you're worried, check the chapter for your child's disorder in Part II, where you'll find information on the accepted treatments.

> **first-line treatment:** The type of treatment tried first for a certain condition or disorder, because it is the most effective and well tolerated.
>
> **second-line treatment:** A type of treatment reserved for use when the first-line treatment is ineffective or not tolerated.

Whether a red flag comes up depends also on who the prescriber is, how well he or she knows your child, how long he or she has been treating your child, what else has been tried first, and whether the diagnosis was made correctly.

I'm inclined to go with my doctor's recommendation for medications, but my husband thinks Tyler doesn't have a real problem—he just needs more discipline. How do we decide who's right?

This is a common dilemma related to a number of points: the parents' perception of the child, the parents' observation of the child, who spends more time and when with the child, the parents' own upbringing and role models, the discipline each parent brings to the child (such as overly strict mother, overly lax father, or vice versa), the specific chemistry or good-ness-of-fit between parent and child, and the presence of a psychiatric dis-order in a parent (who may be more inclined to recognize a similar prob-lem in the child).

On page 36 I explained some of the reasons that it is so difficult to distinguish between a true behavioral disorder and a different kind of problem. These are problems that a professional should be able to sur-mount, but it is not so easy for a lay person. Unfortunately, disagreement between parents over this issue is common and, I'm afraid, potentially harmful to the whole family. One case immediately comes to mind as an il-lustration.

Mrs. Rose brought 9-year-old Sarah into our clinic because Sarah was not listening to her parents or teacher, was hitting other children, being mean to her baby brother, and having bad temper tantrums. Mrs. Rose noted that her daughter did not respond to requests from either parent and said they had been "yelling a lot at Sarah lately" and felt guilty about this. Now both parents were "at the end of their rope." Her sister's kids were all doing well and, similarly, her friends' children did not seem to have any major behavioral or neurological problems. There was one youn-ger son who was doing well. Her marriage was described as "rocky" with some recent strife reported, which was in large part related to their daughter's acting out. Apparently, Mr. Rose, who was from a large family with a strict upbringing, thought that Mrs. Rose needed to be tougher and more consistent in disciplining Sarah. A daughter of an alcoholic father from a smaller family, Mrs. Rose thought that Sarah needed more encour-agement and understanding. Mrs. Rose saw many of her alcoholic father's behaviors in her daughter. Conflicted, Mrs. Rose viewed Sarah's behav-iors as being at times willful and "behavioral" and at other times out of her control.

Mrs. Rose had attended special parenting classes when her daughter was 3 as well as joined a support group for parents of elementary-age stu-dents. She had also received a number of differing opinions about her daughter's problems. Mrs. Rose's mother repeatedly told her that her granddaughter's "naughty behavior" was a result of a lack of love. Her child's school saw it as a discipline problem. Mrs. Rose's sister thought that she was simply too lax in disciplining her daughter when Sarah was acting up. Mrs. Rose's best friend thought that the marital strife was being "thrust" upon the child, and Mr. Rose simply wanted the situation "fixed," because "that's my wife's job." Mrs. Rose believed she was an inadequate parent. She had had a "crazy" father and distant mother herself and supposed that, in part, she had not had proper role models as parents. She was sure that she was making mistakes rearing Sarah, which were adding to her daughter's problems.

Clearly, Mrs. Rose had many opinions on which to draw her conclusion. As strange or paradoxical as it may seem, families are often confrontive and nonsupportive about behavioral issues. Often each member of the extended family has a unique view of the faults of the parents fueling the child's behavior. Family members seem to see it as their obligation to make their opinions known to the parents and are often slow to change their views. As you would expect, family perceptions are based strongly on their own upbringing and experiences. Parents who were raised in discipline-oriented families tend to employ a similar style of child rearing. Conversely, parents from families with a less strict upbringing, or those in whom a family member suffers from mental illness, tend to be more likely to blame an underlying problem in the child or a system in which the child is participating (i.e., school, peers).

Unfortunately, even after I have diagnosed children with a major illness, many families are reluctant to accept that the child's behavior is really related to the illness such as Tourette's disorder and not the parenting. Family members may feel guilty about "passing on the problem" or about being powerless in the situation. They may also exaggerate problematic interactions they have experienced with your child(ren). Since extended family members are often seeing or hearing about your family and child "through the grapevine," they may also be basing their opinions on frank misinformation. Changing the style and perceptions the extended family has about your family and child can be difficult and time-consuming but nevertheless is important and eminently achievable. Persistence and education about your child's problems are the most effective agents. Certainly, family-based therapies can be invaluable to your immediate family not only in educating you about what is wrong with your child but also in identifying and changing family patterns that may have developed as a result of, or are exacerbating, your child's behavior.

Another stress that a difficult child can bring to the family is disruption in the relationship between caregivers. Often the child's primary caregiver and the caregiver's significant other are split over the management of the child. It *is* common that one parent empathizes with the child, perceiving disturbing behaviors as ramifications of a problem. The significant other (or other family members) often sees the picture differently, viewing the child's behavior as manipulative, requiring more discipline.

Commonly both are partially correct; however, these differences often lead to friction between caregivers. It is helpful for both caregivers to feel involved in the process and mutually supported. One of the keys is to work at being unified and supportive of each other. Often to achieve this, scheduled time together, including some downtime, is very effective. For those who are stuck in their ways (entrenched), or in whom preexisting issues are further exacerbated by their children, couples counseling can be invaluable.

None of this is to say that your husband and Mr. Rose are never correct, or partially so. Bad parenting can in fact lead to behavioral and emotional problems that are amenable to treatment. For instance, I treat a number of children who have been physically or sexually abused as younger children who manifest posttraumatic stress disorder (PTSD) and have disabling anxiety. Conversely, an innately psychiatrically disturbed child can destabilize parenting, which in turn further fuels the difficulties in the children. For example, data on the children of substance-abusing parents indicate that, in addition to those children having higher rates of psychiatric problems, they are less resistant to discipline and more difficult to rear. These behaviors in the children, coupled with parents who are substance abusers (many of whom are in recovery and have their own issues), lead to an explosive situation. The solution in these cases is the treatment of the child's behavioral and emotional difficulties *and* parent support or therapy. In our psychopharmacology clinic, in the majority of cases, children have received both medication and therapy, and parents have often engaged in parent support or therapy—alone or with the family.

Unfortunately, some practitioners fail to understand the balance of the child, parents, and family and see all as parenting. Such practitioners fulfill the old adage "If all you have is a hammer, everything looks like a nail." I have encountered a number of both well-meaning and entitled individuals in my own practice who have steadfastly held that the whole issue in the child's behavior is parenting. For example, I treat an adopted 10-year-old boy with depression and conduct disorder who has been raised in a very caring family. His previous provider did not believe in labeling children and on many occasions told the family that the child's shortcomings were based on the child's fantasy of being reunited with the biological parents coupled with the adoptive parents' true love of their biological children. The provider was uninterested in the psychiatric problems of the biological parents (sociopathy and drug abuse in the father). After a formal diagnostic workup, it was found that in addition to depression and conduct disorder, the child had a marked reading difficulty. The boy is doing better now that treatment with Zoloft and clonidine has been started, is receiving assistance for reading, and, with his parents, is involved in behavioral modification. In this case, the specific diagnoses were helpful in explaining the behaviors and focusing treatment.

Our daughter is so young and seems so fragile. How do we know her little body can handle drugs that seem to have such powerful effects?

Certain laboratory tests may be ordered prior to starting medication to ensure that your child's body will handle the medication predictably (see Part III). Included in screening tests for various medications are liver and kidney tests and an electrocardiogram (ECG or EKG). Some medications such as Ritalin or Prozac do not require blood tests, whereas others such as imipramine or lithium will require an EKG.

   The additional testing of these psychotropic drugs in children is also giving us new information on the best dosage range of these medications for younger kids. For example, our group recently published a paper with the manufacturer of Prozac indicating that only 10 mg a day should be started in younger children, as that is the equivalent to 20 mg in an adolescent or adult. In the past, many children were started on the higher dosage. No problems resulting from the administration of that higher dosage were reported, but now we know that only 10 mg a day may be needed. This kind of research finding, as simple as it is, is changing the way doctors are prescribing and should reassure parents that we are all committed to using the least invasive treatment we can find that's effective for children.

> **ECG:** Electrocardiogram, a painless procedure that produces a sketch of the electrical activity of the heart. Also called an *EKG*.

How do I know the recommended drugs are safe?

As you will see throughout this book, despite medications being used commonly for a number of disorders, there is a relative lack of information on the clear effectiveness or safety of certain agents or combinations of medicines for the treatment of childhood disorders. Whereas there are now over 250 scientifically controlled studies of the stimulant medications for ADHD, there are only a handful of studies of medications for juvenile-onset depression or bipolar disorders.

Fortunately, many years of use and a rich clinical experience suggest the safety, tolerability, and usefulness of psychotropics in children. Children should be exposed to a novel medication only if the traditional agents prove ineffective. As is the case with any medication, side effects and adverse reactions can occur. For this reason, it is imperative to understand thoroughly what condition *is* being treated and what *is* the natural history or course of the condition if left untreated. Many of the conditions addressed in this book, such as depression, leave children with high levels of impairment (*morbidity*) and risk of death (*mortality*). Therefore the risk of the medication balances against the benefits of treating the underlying condition.

> **side effect**: An adverse reaction to a treatment that accompanies the effect for which a medication is prescribed. Side effects can either be predictable, such as tiredness, or idiosyncratic, such as liver problems.
>
> **positive effect**: A beneficial outcome of a treatment—the anticipated effect for which a medication is prescribed.

Your practitioner should determine the appropriateness—certainly including safety—of a medication for your child based on information from conferences, published scientific literature, textbooks, consultations, discussions with other providers, the practitioner's own experience, and the experiences of adults with similar disturbances. More recently, bulletin boards with the sole purpose of sharing information on the use of psychotropics in children and teenagers have begun to appear on the Internet, but be careful, since misinformation is plentiful.

Information obtained from systematic observations either through careful review of medical records or controlled clinical trials constitutes the most authentic information on which to base clinical practice. In the absence of such information, discussions of a medication or combination of medications with my colleagues is important to me in deciding what compounds to use in the care of my own patients.

> **clinical trial:** A systematic and scientific evaluation of a new treatment for a disorder.

In fact, it is not unusual for prescribers to rely on their own clinical experience. Often, practitioners will continue to use an agent that is reported in the scientific literature to have no effect for the purpose prescribed—such as the use of nortriptyline as the only treatment (monotherapy) for an anxiety disorder when they have observed success in their own practice. Or they may combine drugs, knowing that certain medications (such as nortriptyline) treat specific symptoms of a disorder.

Rest assured that prescribers are much more sophisticated about the armamentarium of psychotropics as well as the necessities of a careful diagnostic evaluation than they were in the past. Some prescribers still tend to go directly to the "big guns" such as the antipsychotics for behavioral problems (such as use of Risperdal as a first agent for ADHD), and this practice should not be condoned. Fortunately, I have seen a vast reduction in misuse of medications by prescribers over the past 5 years.

Keep in mind, too, that many of the SSRIs are now approved for adolescents with a variety of conditions (mainly obsessive–compulsive disorder); Strattera for ADHD in children, adolescents, and adults; and Risperdal is soon to be FDA-approved for children and adolescents with "disruptive disorders" (oppositional and conduct disorder). The approval process is ongoing, so new drugs are receiving approval for various conditions all the time.

Concern remains, however, about the effects of long-term use of these agents in children. In Parts II and III of this book I'll tell you everything we know to date about the long-term risks associated with each medication. But the fact is that long-term studies are extremely difficult to conduct. Not only do you have to recruit a very large group of children into the study, but they typically have to stay on one medication (or one treatment) for a number of years. Life is simply not that simple: kids move away, get tired of being in a study, or their treatment is changed (or they just stop their treatment). Fortunately, the data we do have are positive. For example, despite the use of SSRIs in children for over a decade, no long-term side effects have emerged in the literature or in case reports. In contrast, probably the most problematic long-term effects will be associated with the atypical antipsychotics such as Zyprexa and Risperdal—largely because of their effects on increasing weight and potential effects on metabolism; see Chapter 17 for details.

One finding you should be aware of is that recent reanalysis of large datasets of some SSRIs has brought to our attention the rare occurrence of the emergence of fleeting suicidal thoughts (coincidentally, no harm in any of the trials was reported). While some SSRIs have been found under controlled conditions (vs. placebo) to be effective for depression (e.g., Prozac) and others have failed that test (Effexor, Paxil), the FDA and manufacturers have recommended that Paxil and Effexor not be used for child or adolescent depression until they have sorted out the complicated issue regarding a link between the drugs and suicide. Having said that, it is important to keep in context that no serious suicidality was reported with either medication, and clinical use of these compounds for almost a decade has suggested an important role for these medications in the portfolio of available treatments for depression. Nevertheless, close observation of your child during the early phases of treatment (6 weeks) for problematic side effects such as fleeting suicidal thoughts is warranted *on all medications* for depression.

Isn't caution justified, considering everything I've read in newspapers and magazines and seen on TV about overuse and misuse of these medicines?

If you have any concerns at all about what you have heard about a medication prescribed for your child, discuss them with the pharmacist and/or the child's doctor. If you have placed your trust in these professionals before, trusting them now is probably a good bet. Misinformation is a fact of life in psychiatry and medicine just as it is in many other fields, and sometimes myths are hard to dispel. How a comment becomes established as "fact" often depends on the emotion-laden environment, intelligence of the readers, nature of the data, and conviction of the reporter.

Unfortunately some myths continue to influence clinical practice. For example, there is little data to support that Ritalin worsens or causes seizures; in fact, the most recent studies clearly dispute those findings. However, that concern is still listed in the *Physicians' Desk Reference (PDR),* a compendium of information on brand name and generic prescription medications currently available. Likewise, there is no information that children's exposure to medication will transform them into drug addicts in young adulthood, but many parents still fear this outcome. Actually, a robust collection of current research findings suggests that the underlying disorder for which the child is being treated is the major risk factor for later problems with alcohol or drugs.

One caveat: Be cautious about the medication *du jour* that may appear on the Internet. Increasingly, parents download information from a variety of sources on specific medications, some of which is frankly wrong and much of which is not referenced. Be extremely cautious in accepting this information as gospel. There are no standards governing Internet information, so always check the data and the source. Your best bet is to rely only on websites sponsored by dependable nonprofit sources such as the American Academy of Pediatrics or the American Academy of Child and Adolescent Psychiatry (see "Resources"). More recently, the pharmaceutical industry has developed websites about its medications that are another good source of more specific information.

Most clinicians will be a comprehensive and honest source of information on the drugs they prescribe. I, for one, believe that an informed parent is a more effective partner in the treatment of the child, and so I attempt to answer all questions about drug safety with total candor.

I looked up the drug my child's doctor wants to prescribe and found that it's not FDA-approved for use in children. Shouldn't I refuse to let my son take it?

Your child's doctor is obligated to discuss any major risks of the medication with you but will not necessarily discuss the status of U.S. Food and Drug Administration (FDA) approval of the drug with you. Please don't conclude that this indicates dishonesty or secrecy on the doctor's part. As a clinical researcher, I am involved in a number of trials of experimental medications, some of which are going to be submitted to the FDA for approval. The process of FDA approval is quite complicated, cumbersome, and lengthy. Practitioners do not have to discuss FDA status; they do, however, have to discuss the risks of the medication.

Why do most inserts and descriptions of the medications in the *PDR* say that they are "Not recommended for use in children"? The majority of medications employed in child psychiatry have been approved for use in adults, but have not been studied extensively by the pharmaceutical industry in children. For example, despite common use in this country, medications such as clonidine or desipramine for ADHD, lithium for mood problems in youth, and even Ritalin in preschoolers are not FDA-approved in these age groups. FDA approval means that the government has carefully reviewed the studies on the effectiveness and tolerability of the medications and has deemed that the medication can be marketed for a specific disorder in a specified age group. The lack of FDA approval does not preclude the use of any given psychoactive medication in children (or any other group). The age limit on any FDA-approved drug—such as Luvox, approved only for those 8 years and older—means generally that the testers did not study the use of the drug in a younger group. The use of the medications in other groups of individuals is not necessarily dangerous but simply has not been studied and therefore has not received the FDA "stamp of approval." It is important to note that in the practice of medicine clinicians frequently use medications for reasons not specifically addressed in FDA guidelines (a good example is aspirin for prevention of heart attacks).

PDR entries include only uses for which the drug can be marketed or advertised. For example, all of the new serotonin-specific antidepressants have been used and appear effective for obsessive–compulsive disorders in children; however, only Luvox and Zoloft (sertraline) are formally approved by the FDA and hence are the only ones indicated for this condition in advertisements and in the *PDR*. Note, too, that although safe for use in children suffering from anxiety or depression, Luvox and Zoloft are not FDA-approved for that use. So, FDA approval is more complicated— and more limited—than it may seem. It is important to point out, however, that the FDA monitors serious problems arising from medication use, through voluntary physician reporting. Based on its review of such problems, the FDA sends physician alerts about the possibility of medication-related problems.

If these drugs don't need FDA approval to be used in kids like mine, how are they tested for safety and effectiveness?

As mentioned earlier (page 22), doctors know that the drugs are effective for the use prescribed mainly from clinical evidence—information obtained from the actual practice of medicine. Clinical evidence may include data from studies performed in human subjects or experience derived from day-to-day practice. Studies performed to determine whether a medication works in people involve asking general and specific questions of patients, checking their vital signs and doing blood tests, and sometimes testing how their brains are working.

Most of what we know about medications comes from two types of investigations: open studies and placebo-controlled trials. Both types of studies are based on knowing what is wrong with the child (diagnosis) and carefully observing the child through the study to determine if the medication works (*efficacy*) and if there are side effects. An *open study* is a trial in which both the patient/family and the doctor are aware of the study medication being used. An example would be having a child on a specific drug for a given disorder with weekly monitoring for 6 weeks. At each visit, the child and parents (and sometimes teachers) are asked questions and rated as to how the medication is working, the child has his blood pressure and pulse checked, and the doctor asks about side effects. Often, there will be a long-term open phase of a study that follows immediately after a controlled investigation (see below), mainly to assess for safety concerns over time.

In the more relied-on and accurate controlled trials, the use of an inert substance referred to as *a placebo* is employed. Despite years of trying to tease out a placebo response, the scientific community still does not know why some individuals respond to an inactive compound. There is no specific personality type that responds or does not respond to a placebo. In a placebo-controlled study, the placebo and active medication tablets or capsules appear identical.

> **placebo:** An inactive compound such as sugar pills, used in scientific studies to determine how much of a medication's positive effect comes from the medication and how much from other factors, such as seeing the doctor frequently.

To further eliminate bias from the study, in some studies, the child, parent, doctor, or some combination may not know if the child is taking a placebo or the active medication. This purposeful attempt to mask whether the child is receiving active medication is referred to as a *blind*. If both the child/parent and doctor are unaware if the child is receiving the active medication or placebo, the trial is referred to as a *double-blind study*. You can see that by using this mechanism you can eliminate the bias of unconsciously having a response based on receiving the active medication.

In some type of studies referred to as *parallel design,* a child will receive either the active medication or the placebo throughout the study. In contrast, in a *cross-over* investigation, the child will receive both placebo and active medication at different points in the study. The overall response is roughly derived from subtracting the response of the children receiving placebo from the response of those receiving the active medication being tested. As you can imagine, these controlled trials can cost millions of dollars, are labor-intensive, and often take from 3 to 5 years to complete. Often they are conducted simultaneously at multiple sites throughout the country.

How can the drug our doctor wants to prescribe be "safe" when the PDR lists about a dozen scary side effects?

The *PDR* overly lists side effects observed in individuals who have taken this drug in clinical trials and in reports after the medication is on the market. Most people will not experience any of these side effects. You can also take comfort in the fact that, as a rule, prescribers will begin treating children with the lowest possible dose of a drug to get the most positive effect with the least side effects. Remember, however, that there is no such thing as a drug with no side effects. Even though your child will be taking the medicine as treatment for a "brain disorder," the whole body will be bathed by the medication as the drug circulates through the child's bloodstream. The major area in which Zoloft and Prozac work, for example, is the brain, yet they circulate throughout the body, including the stomach and intestines, and that is why they may cause cramps and diarrhea.

With all these safety and side-effect issues to consider, exactly how does a doctor decide which drug to prescribe?

The doctor decides on a drug—and every other aspect of your child's treatment—on the basis of the risk–benefit ratio involved in using that treatment. The practitioner will compare all the benefits of the treatment—the improvements in symptoms that the drug should produce and the future damage that may be prevented by treating the child now—with the risks, or side effects, of taking the drug. If the benefits outweigh the risks, the doctor may decide to prescribe that drug for your child. How great the ratio must be in favor of the benefits depends to some extent on how severe the impairments that your child and family are suffering because of the child's disorder.

Yet, side effects don't always have to be seen as the enemy. Practitioners decide to use specific medications in part *because* of their side effects. For example, your doctor may choose to use a medication with more sedative properties to be given at night if your child is having prominent sleep problems. Conversely, children who are withdrawn or low in energy may benefit from a medication that stimulates the child's energy, often reducing sedation. Following these guidelines in depressed children, for example, might lead to the use of Prozac or Paxil in low-energy children and Luvox for those with difficulty falling asleep. Some medicines, such as nortriptyline for ADHD, may be associated with weight gain and can be helpful in underweight children. Medicines like Topamax (topirimate) and Kepra (levetiracetam) are being used by practitioners because they lead to weight loss—an important antidote to some of the effective agents we use for Tourette's disorder, psychosis, and bipolar disorder that cause significant weight gain in children.

Other medications such as the Prozac-like medications (Lexapro, Celexa, Zoloft, Luvox, Paxil) or the stimulants (Ritalin, Dexedrine, Cylert, Metadate, Adderall, and Concerta) can benefit overweight children because they are associated with either no weight change or actual weight loss. Strattera, a new medication for ADHD, may be useful for kids with sleep problems associated with their ADHD.In choosing a medication, then, the doctor will look for one whose side effects can be seen as benefits rather than risks.

---

sedative: Sleep-producing.

Has the doctor made a mistake? The dosage recommended for my 11-year-old daughter is the same amount my adult cousin is taking.

If you have any doubts at all about dosage, ask the doctor and then double-check with a pharmacist you trust. Generally, though, children require more medication given their size compared to adults because they are more efficient in breaking down and eliminating medications. (An exception, our group discovered, is Prozac, as mentioned on page 224.) In addition, children may have more severe illness and multiple disorders. Finally, some medications, such as lithium, are relatively weak (but effective) and require higher doses to work.

The younger you are, the more quickly your body breaks down drugs, making them inactive and/or ready for elimination. This means more of a drug is needed to treat a given problem. This fact explains why some infant formulas of over-the-counter (OTC) drugs are actually more concentrated than the child versions, a fact that has caused some parents to overdose their older children unwittingly.

> **OTC:** Over the counter; available without a
> prescription.

The two major organs involved in the breakdown (metabolism or ca-
tabolism) of medications are the liver (hepatic system) and kidneys (renal
system). Lithium and Neurontin are broken down by the kidneys and excreted in the urine, but the majority of psychoactive medications—including the antidepressants, anxiety-breaking medications, anticonvulsants,
atomoxetine, and stimulants—are broken down by the liver and are
passed out of the body in the stool.

> **stimulants:** A class of medications—including
> methylphenidate (Ritalin), amphetamines (Dexedrine,
> Adderall), and pemoline (Cylert)—thought to activate
> the central nervous system.

Because children tend to metabolize their medications about twice as
fast as adults, it is not uncommon for a typical adult to require 150 mg of
imipramine and for his 12-year-old son to require the same dose. It is also
not unusual for a child to lose a response to a previously helpful medication, in part because the child is growing but the tablet size is not. Conversely, you may be able to reduce the dose of a medication as your
daughter grows simply because her metabolism is beginning to slow down
and she no longer requires as much medication.

How do prescribers determine an appropriate dosage?

Doctors determine doses of medication based on safety, strength, and effectiveness of the compound. How well a medication works or, more technically, the amount of change the medication causes in the symptoms of a
disorder is called its *efficacy,* or *effectiveness.* The amount of medication it
takes to get a response indicates how strong the drug is and is referred to
as *potency.* (A good analogy is to gasoline: 93-octane gas is more potent
than 87-octane.) Your child will require lower doses of more potent medication (such as Haldol) and higher doses of a lower-potency agent (such as
Thorazine). One confusing point, however: It is common for two medications to be roughly equal in how they will work (efficacy). However, it
may take different amounts of the medications to get a similar response
(potency). The antidepressant agents offer a good illustration of this point.

Whereas your depressed child may require only 20 mg of Prozac, she would need approximately 100–150 mg of Zoloft to have the same effect. Similarly, 100 mg of desipramine is roughly equivalent (*equipotent*) to 50 mg of nortriptyline or 25 mg of protriptyline. With the antipsychotic medications, 1–2 mg of Haldol is roughly equivalent to 100 mg of Thorazine. In each of these cases, the medications have about the *same* ability to treat the problem (efficacy); however, different amounts are necessary (potency) due to their chemical composition. It is also noteworthy that side effects are specific for each medication and that 20 mg of Prozac has roughly similar amounts of side effects to 100 mg of Zoloft. Therefore each medication has specific properties that determine how effective and strong it is for a specific disorder, and this "rating" typically differs among medications.

Because children vary so widely in body size, doctors often determine dosing of certain compounds such as Strattera (atomoxetine) or the tricyclic antidepressants (desipramine, nortriptyline, and imipramine) by the child's body weight, usually expressed via the metric system: milligrams of medication per kilogram of body weight (mg per kg). Table 3 shows the typical dosing of the bulk of medications used for emotional and behavioral disorders in children and adolescents. When using this table, remember that 1 kg = 2.2 pounds. A 110-pound adolescent, for example, weighs about 50 kg, and for that child a typical dose of Strattera would be 60 mg, or 1.2 mg per kilogram of the child's weight.

In large part because of side effects, psychotropics are started at the lowest possible dose. Your doctor may ask you to increase the medication to a specific dose at some point in time and to increase the medication every so often until your child has a positive response, cannot tolerate the medication because of side effects, or has reached the maximum amount suggested by the doctor.

Although many dosages will be determined by the child's weight, there is often an amount of medication that an individual your child's age usually requires on a regular day-to-day basis. For example, it is common for doctors to use from 18 to 72 mg of Concerta per dose in a typical school-age child.

How will the doctor determine whether the dosage is correct once my child starts taking the medication?

As you will learn in more detail in the section "Treatment and Beyond," there are various ways to monitor the effects of your child's medication. To

TABLE 3. Typical Pediatric Dosages of Psychotropic Drugs

Medication	Daily dose	Weight-adjusted daily dose*	Daily dosage schedule
Stimulants			
Dextro-amphetamine/ amphetamine compounds	5–60 mg	0.3–1.5 mg/kg	Two or three times (once for extended-release forms)
Methylphenidate	5–90 mg	1.0–2.0 mg/kg	Two or three times (once for extended-release forms)
D-Methylphenidate	2.5–45 mg	0.5–1.0 mg/kg	Two or three times (once for extended-release forms)
Magnesium pemoline	37.5–150 mg	1.0–3.0 mg/kg	One or two times
Atomoxetine	18–100 mg	0.5–1.2 mg/kg	One or two times
Antidepressants			
Tricyclics (TCAs) Imipramine Desipramine Amitriptyline Nortriptyline Clomipramine	10–300 mg	2.0–5.0 mg/kg (0.5–3.0 mg/kg for nortriptyline and protriptyline); dose adjusted according to response and serum levels	One or two times
Selective serotonin reuptake inhibitors (SSRIs)			
Fluoxetine	5–40 mg	0.25–0.70 mg/kg	One or two times
Sertraline	25–200 mg	1.5–3.0 mg/kg	
Paroxetine	10–30 mg	0.25–0.70 mg/kg	
Fluvoxamine	50–300 mg	1.5–4.5 mg/kg	
(Es)Citalopram	5–40 mg	0.25–0.70 mg/kg	
Atypical			
Bupropion	37.5–400 mg	3–6 mg/kg	Three times
Venlafaxine	25–150 mg	1–3 mg/kg	Two or three times
Nefazodone	50–400 mg	1–8 mg/kg	Two times
Trazodone	50–200 mg	2–4 mg/kg	Two times

(cont.)

TABLE 3. *(continued)*

Medication	Daily dose	Weight-adjusted daily dose*	Daily dosage schedule
Antipsychotics			

Phenothiazines
  Low potency
  (e.g., Mellaril,
  Thorazine,
  Clozaril, Seroquel)
	25–400 mg	3–6 mg/kg	One or two generally
			One to three times

Medium potency
  (e.g., Navane,
  Trilafon, Stelazine,
  Geodon, Zyprexa)
	5–60 mg	1–3 mg/kg	

High potency
  (e.g., Prolixin,
  Haldol, Orap,
  Risperidal)
	0.5–20 mg	0.1–0.5 mg/kg	

Medications to reduce mania in bipolar disorder			
Lithium carbonate	300–2,100 mg	10–30 mg/kg (use levels)	One or two times
Valproate	250–1,500 mg	15–60 mg/kg (use levels)	Two times
Carbamazepine	200–1,000 mg	10–20 mg/kg (use levels)	Two times with meals
Gabapentin	300–1,200 mg	10 mg/kg	Three times
Lamotrigine	50–200 mg	1–3 mg/kg	Two times
Topamax	50–400 mg	3–6 mg/kg	Two times
Gabitril	4–32 mg	0.1–1 mg/kg	Two times
Trileptal	300–1,200 mg	10–20 mg/kg	Two times

(cont.)

TABLE 3. (continued)

Medication	Daily dose	Weight-adjusted daily dose*	Daily dosage schedule
Antianxiety medications			
Buspirone	5–45 mg	0.5–1.0 mg/kg	Three times
High-potency benzodiazepines			
Klonopin (long–acting)	0.5–6 mg	0.02–0.10 mg/kg	One or two times
Xanax (short-acting)	0.5–6 mg	0.02–0.10 mg/kg	Three times
Ativan (short-acting)	0.5–6 mg	0.04–0.15 mg/kg	Three times
Lower-potency diazepines			
Valium, Tranxene	3.75–30 mg	0.1–1 mg/kg	Three times
Antihypertensives			
Clonidine	0.025–0.6 mg	3–10 µg	Two to four times and at bedtime
Guanfacine	0.25–4 mg	.02–0.10 mg/kg Two or three times	
Propranolol	20–240 mg	2–8 mg/kg	Two times
Other			
Naltrexone	25–75 mg	1–2 mg/kg	Two or three times
Desmopressin (ddAVP)	One to two times nightly	3–10 µg (0.1–0.2 ml)	Intranasal; one or two times
	0.2–0.6 mg	Not applicable	One to three tablets at bedtime

*To calculate your child's body weight in kilograms (kg), divide his or her weight in pounds by 2.2.

state it simply, the best way to determine whether the dosage is too high or too low is to observe the child. If your child's condition has improved as expected but side effects are bothersome, you and the doctor may want to consider a slightly lower dose. If there are no side effects but improvement is also minimal, you may want to try increasing the dose a bit.

The other common method for monitoring dosage is blood tests. Tests of the blood levels of a medication can reveal whether your child is taking the medication in the first place (*adherence*), as well as whether the dose is high enough to begin causing toxicity in the form of side effects or too low to be effective. Blood tests can also identify children—about 1 in 10—who are particularly slow at breaking down medications. Because these slow metabolizers will end up with high concentrations of the compound in their blood, prescribers usually order blood tests for some medications, notably antidepressants and anticonvulsants, when first starting treatment. Similarly, blood tests are important when children are taking more than one medication because some drugs interact and slow each other's metabolism. Prozac, for example, used to treat children with depression, markedly reduces the breakdown of desipramine, used to treat ADHD. So, children being treated with these drugs for both disorders can end up with very high levels of desipramine in their blood. *Always discuss possible drug interactions with all of your child's doctors.* Mental health providers need to know about all drugs your child is taking, because psychotropic drugs can interact with even over-the-counter drugs. Your child's other doctors need to know about psychotropic prescriptions, especially if they want to start your child on a medicine such as Acutane for acne, or an antibiotic for an infection.

> **blood level:** The amount or concentration of medication in the blood. Also called *serum* or *plasma concentration.*
>
> **drug interaction:** A change in the concentration and effectiveness of a drug when administered along with another drug. One medication can increase or decrease the usefulness of another.

For all of these reasons, each child will have a different amount of medication that actually makes its way to the brain to reduce the symptoms of the disorder, and no simple blood or other test will reveal the exact dosage that is appropriate for that child. Be prepared for an adjustment period.

Why does my child have to take three drugs instead of one?

It may be comforting to know that multiple agents are being used increasingly in both clinical practice and research for the treatment of child and adolescent psychiatric disorders, as well as in the practice of medicine in general. Doctors use combined pharmacotherapy for the following reasons: (1) co-occurring disorders (comorbidity, such as depression plus anxiety); (2) inadequate response to a single agent (adding Klonopin to Paxil is common in kids with panic disorder); (3) synergism between two medications (such as desipramine and Adderall for ADHD); and (4) the need to treat the side effects of an effective medication (such as use of Cogentin to reduce muscle spasms caused by Haldol).

> **comorbid**: Occurring at the same time as another problem or disorder.

Multiple drugs are often prescribed so that your child can get the greatest effect with the least side effects. Doses of one drug that would be large enough to completely treat a given disorder may sometimes result in intolerable adverse effects. For example, in children with ADHD, the dosage of Ritalin necessary for satisfactory control of ADHD may lead to poor appetite, edginess, staring spells, and insomnia. However, the combination of Dexedrine and low-dose nortriptyline may lead to a better response, while eliminating the wear-off and side effects caused by the Dexedrine. Likewise, anxious children often require both an antidepressant compound such as Zoloft and a Valium-like agent to break panic and anxiety problems. Children who have prominent mood swings despite the use of hefty doses of mood stabilizers such as Depakote, Trileptal, Neurontin, Lamictal, or lithium often gain a substantial reduction in mood swings from using the mood stabilizers together. For instance, a 17-year-old boy with bipolar mood disorder receiving modest doses of Depakote (1,500 mg daily) had a marginal improvement in his mood but continued to have periodic outbursts resulting in suspensions from school and home problems. The addition of 300 mg twice daily of lithium resulted in a marked reduction in his mood swings (*lability*), and over time we were able to reduce his Depakote to 1,000 mg daily with continued good control of his mood and less sedation caused by the Depakote. Besides the medications Cogentin, Artane, and Amantadine, commonly prescribed to take care of the muscular spasms caused by antipsychotics, the beta-blockers, of which propanolol is the most well known, are sometimes used for the edginess associated with the stimulant class of medications. Similarly, Remeron (mirtazapine) or Catapres (clonidine) is prescribed at the hour of sleep to treat the insomnia caused by the stimulants or other agents.

A number of issues need to be taken into consideration when combining agents. Despite this common practice, there is generally a lack of scientific studies demonstrating the effectiveness and safety of using two or more agents simultaneously. When combining medications, be aware that it is harder to remember to give all of the medications at the times specified. Along the same lines, your child will not like having to take additional medications, making compliance even more difficult. You should ask about potential drug-to-drug interactions that may arise between or among the agents to be used as well as with OTC medications. Interactions with atomoxetine or the Prozac-like family of antidepressants need to be considered. Finally, cost may be a factor, since two or more medications may cost more than a single agent, especially if you have to copay $5–20 (or more) per monthly prescription.

Don't the many interactions among drugs make timing the dosages paramount? What if we don't stick perfectly to the schedule?

Whether your child is taking one drug or several, timing of doses is not nearly as important as being sure that your child is actually taking the medication. Except for the short-acting stimulants and Valium-like medications, parents can move the administration time of medications around to optimize response (after-school dosing of Tegretol), improve compliance (giving once-daily medication instead of three times a day), and reduce side effects or use them to the child's benefit (administering sedating imipramine before bedtime). In general, few medicines need to be given at precise times. However, your child will be more compliant using a routine or a schedule. Medications given once a day are certainly easier to remember—think of your own difficulties in remembering to take four-per-day antibiotics—but if your child has to take medicine more often, spread them out as well as you can according to your family's schedule. Three-times-a-day medication does not have to be taken at exact 8-hour intervals; giving the medication at breakfast, lunch, and dinner is usually quite acceptable. Most of the medications used for behavioral and emotional disorders can be given with meals, which not only makes it easier to remember but often results in fewer side effects. In particular, drugs such as Tegretol and lithium are much better tolerated when given with meals.

Drugs that are more activating in nature, such as stimulants or certain antidepressants (such as Wellbutrin or Prozac), are generally given in the morning. Medications used to treat daytime anxiety or ADHD should also be given just prior to or with breakfast. Agents that may cause tiredness are often given at night and can be given with dinner or before your child's bedtime. Medicines given "at hour of sleep" should be given approximately one hour prior to the expected bedtime and with a snack.

After a new medicine or combination of agents is begun, be sure to observe closely to learn the major and subtle effects on your child. With this information, your child's practitioner can work with you to reduce bothersome side effects. For example, a 14-year-old girl that I treat wanted to stop taking her Zoloft, despite the fact that it was alleviating her depression, because it was also making her fall asleep in class. Simply switching to taking the whole dose at dinner solved the problem.

Inevitably your child will miss a dose of medication. Generally a missed dose is not a problem. If you plan to give a missed dose the next day (such as a bedtime antidepressant given in the morning), be aware that your child may be tired during school. More problematic is giving your child the medication twice. Inadvertent double dosing is generally not dangerous, but it may create a problem and should be discussed with the pharmacist or your doctor. Most pharmacies provide a printout on the medication that includes contingencies for missed or double doses. You should also be aware of what medications can be held (not given) if your child is ill. Children who are nauseated or vomiting may not tolerate certain agents, and it may be advisable to hold single doses of the medication (such as lithium, Wellbutrin, and stimulants).

Will my child become tolerant to the medication?

One of the most perplexing issues in pediatric psychopharmacology is the development of tolerance to medications. Although not a problem for the majority of children, an estimated 10–25% do lose the effect of their medication, so it is best to be prepared for the possibility. Having stabilized a child on medication, it can be demoralizing to the child and family to see the effect dissipate. In some cases, the child's problematic behaviors return insidiously.

> **tolerance:** Increasing resistance to a drug resulting from continued use.

If you suspect that your child is losing a response to a medication, contact the doctor and be prepared to discuss what might be causing the problem. First, query your child and do a pill count. If your child is taking the medication, has she started taking other medications or special diet supplements? These could be interfering with the metabolism of the medication. Also consider the possibility that your child is developing another problem such as anxiety and depression. One 13-year-old boy I treat for depression was brought in because his Luvox was not working. An exam showed that he had developed a separate anxiety problem, which responded to the treatment I then prescribed.

> **metabolism:** Ongoing chemical processes that create (*anabolism*) or break down (*catabolism*) compounds.

In cases where your child has lost the effect of the medication, a number of strategies can be tried. An increase in the dosage may be all that is necessary if your child is growing rapidly. The use of low doses of adjunctive agents such as Buspar or lithium may help reclaim the response. Changing to another medication within the same class can also be useful. Studies have shown that Dexedrine or Adderall can be effective in a child who no longer responds to Concerta or Ritalin. Similarly, our group has shown that the majority of kids who lose their response to the stimulants or desipramine will respond to nortriptyline, and vice versa. Children no longer responding to a specific antidepressant or antipsychotic should be tried on another agent within the class.

> **adjunctive agent:** A second drug prescribed to bolster the effectiveness of the first.

Some parents ask about the use of medication "holidays" (see page 135) to prevent tolerance. Outside of Parkinson's disease, there remains scant scientific information to support or reject this practice. You need to carefully balance the real risks of not treating your child against any potentially positive effects of drug holidays.

My doctor keeps going back and forth on choosing my son's prescription. Does he know what he's doing?

A doctor's lack of absolute certainty should not be taken as poor clinical medicine or lack of professional knowledge. In fact, the doctor's willingness to express doubts to you is a good sign that you've found a doctor with whom you can communicate openly. My colleagues and I are all guilty of this ambivalence, in part because psychiatric disorders in children are difficult to diagnose and in part because arriving at the best possible medication regimen is challenging. The fact is trial and error may be the only way to reach the best possible dose and combination of drugs and the best possible balance of psychopharmacology and psychotherapy for your child.

How many medication trials should we expect, and how can we get through them?

It always helps to understand what is to be achieved and to be involved in the process. Parents and their children should take actions to avoid feeling hopeless or helpless during the trial. Try not to focus on each symptom and how the child is doing from hour to hour; instead, attempt a more global appraisal of how things are this week compared to last week.

> **medication trial:** A systematic test of a medication in a patient that usually takes 1–3 months.

The general rule is to use a medication at a reasonable dose (if tolerated) for at least 1 month. Always ensure that the medication is being taken properly (or at all). After two unsuccessful medication trials, reevaluate the diagnosis to ensure that the underpinnings of the treatment are correct. There is no upper limit on when to call it quits with medication for *those* disorders that are known to respond pharmacologically. Remember, untreated, many of these disorders may lead to future problems as the child passes into adulthood.

How will the medication trial affect my child's school life?

The medication trial itself does not necessarily have to affect your child's school life at all. However, if you haven't considered it already, be aware that children with psychiatric disorders often have learning disabilities as well. The psychiatric disorders themselves also may cause academic difficulties. You need to work with your child's school to ensure the best possible education despite these potential obstacles.

If your child is struggling academically, you should be sure that she has had cognitive testing to assess for learning potential (IQ), current fund of knowledge (achievement), or specific learning disabilities. During this period, communication with the school's psychologist can be invaluable. Your child's learning environment may need to be changed to reflect findings from the assessment.

In addition to the psychological testing provided by the school to assess your child's academic and cognitive functioning (including the presence of learning disabilities), you should schedule an educational planning meeting to discuss extra needs your child may have. Generally schools invite parental participation in the process. Facilitate discussion of behavioral management and additional resources that may be available to ensure your child's success.

Informing the school of the ongoing psychiatric care of your child is useful; however, as mentioned earlier in this section, schools tend to adhere to less stringent rules of confidentiality than medical or psychiatric professionals. With the availability of extended-release preparations of medications (Adderall XR, Concerta, Metadate CD, and Ritalin LA, for example) and once-daily nonstimulants (Strattera, Wellbutrin XL, tricyclics), the school does not have to be involved in the administration of the medication for many disorders. If the school requests a comprehensive psychiatric assessment to authenticate your child's diagnosis, I suggest having your doctor write a brief letter specifically addressing the diagnosis, treatment (including medications), and specific educational or behavioral needs. It is a good idea to discuss with your child's practitioner specific remedial needs that should be included in the letter to assist the school in knowing what to include in the educational plan.

> **remedial:** Designed to ameliorate or cure someone's deficits, such as academic problems.

You have the option of accepting or rejecting the educational plan once it is developed. If you are not satisfied, you can request minor changes or an alternative plan. Although not usually necessary, trained advocates are available to work with the school system on behalf of you and your child. Schedule an update session to measure the plan's success about a month after changes are implemented.

Also consider finding an advocate within the school, such as a guidance counselor or teacher, to serve as a vital link among you, your child, and the school. Both you and your child should feel comfortable talking to this person. Your child should have regular contact with him or her and also be able to turn to this person when having a bad day. You should be in close contact with this advocate to get feedback about your child's response to treatment, particularly medication trials. Finally, this advocate should be able to facilitate discussion between you and individual teachers and other school personnel.

What should we tell the school about the upcoming medication trial?

Ideally, you would plan to work especially closely with the school during medication trials, particularly for those disorders such as ADHD that manifest largely in the school setting. Based on your individual school's policy on mental health, you should attempt to receive some form of acceptable feedback on your child's condition. While working within the law and your school's policy on information transfer relative to mental health, you should plan to collect useful information as to your child's response to medication. If possible, establish weekly contacts with the school during the initiation of different pharmacological trials. Some parents tell the school all of the specifics of the trial such as the dose of the medication and expected action and side effects. Others choose only to ask for a report of their child's behavior without mentioning that there is a medication trial under way.

There are pros and cons to both approaches. Keeping the school fully informed makes personnel feel more involved in the process, which in turn tends to make them more collaborative and understanding. It also means you can expect more feedback, including suggestions that you may or may not welcome. In this case, you will have to keep an eye out for teacher biases; some feel strongly that one medication is effective over another, often based on very limited experience. Asking only for weekly reports eliminates this problem but also robs you of possible collaborative input. A compromise might be to let the school know that the child may be receiving a number of different medications and that you will be asking for feedback weekly. This sets up a sort of scientifically blinded trial in which the observer (in this case the teacher) is unaware of the specific medication or dose being employed. If you choose this approach, I strongly suggest communicating your reasons in an attempt to keep the school personnel as collaborators rather than risking an adversarial relationship.

If your child is to receive medications during the school day, the school's nurse will quickly become one of your most important contacts. School nurses (or, in the absence of a nurse, another designated staff member; check with the individual school) are generally responsible for holding and dispensing any medication to be given at school and will play an important role in your child's care. Despite the availability of extended-release stimulants, some children will respond only to short-acting stimulants. The short-acting stimulants such as Dexedrine and Ritalinare are given around lunchtime to cover behaviors in the afternoon, and the school nurse will be in charge of this process. Other medicines, such as clonidine or guanfacine, may also require a lunchtime dose. The nurse can be of great assistance in monitoring your child, giving you feedback on problem side effects and the effectiveness of the medication during the school day. The nurse may also be quite knowledgeable about your child's medication and therefore can be a great source of information. How much communication and assistance you can expect, however, depends on the scope of the nursing staff at the school. Some schools have a staff of full-time nurses, some have only a part-time nurse, and some have no medical personnel at all.

Most schools have a well-worked-out procedure for dispensing medication. Generally state laws dictate that children are not allowed to carry and take their own medications in school. Similarly, schools are usually required to have forms filled out by both your child's physician and you regarding your child's diagnosis and the specifics of dispensing the medication. Many schools will not start giving medications, or change the type or dose of the medications, until these forms are completed and a well-labeled prescription bottle with the medication is brought in by a caregiver. It is a good idea to ask for a couple of extra forms and take them with you to your child's follow-up medication visits in case the medication dose is changed.

Be sure that your child's physician prescribes a large enough quantity of the medication to cover your child both at school and at home. Some schools require a separate bottle of medication with the specific time and dose of medication prescribed for the school hours. Others will allow prescriptions that include other times of administration as long as the required school dosing is specified (this is preferable since it means a copay for only one prescription instead of two). For instance, Focalin (a high-tech form of Ritalin/methylphenidate) is usually prescribed for both a morning and a noon dose: "Give one 5-mg tablet with breakfast and again at noon." This tells the school exactly what dose to give and at what time.

CHAPTER 4

TREATMENT AND BEYOND
Collaborating in Your Child's Ongoing Care

The planning stages are over; now your child is embarking on treatment. Your child may do well with the first drug tried at the initial dosage, or you may have to endure several medication trials before an effective regimen is reached. Either way, as a developing creature, your child will face evolving needs, and you may be wise to expect the unexpected. Keep your powers of observation sharp and the lines of communication open.

Many of the questions I hear about this ongoing phase of the psychopharmacological treatment of children concern the definition of roles: "What can I do to make sure my child continues to do well?" "How much responsibility should my child take for his own care?" "When should I call the doctor?" Everyone who has an interest in your child's continued well-being plays an important part in the proactive measures described in the following pages. Practical details also become important. Do you need to change the child's diet or lifestyle to optimize the treatment effect? Can you use generics as well as brand name drugs? How do you time administration of the drug for the best effect and the fewest side effects? What do you need to know about other prescription drugs and over-the-counter medications? Answers to questions like these can help the whole family adapt to your child's psychopharmacological treatment.

As a parent, what should I be doing now that my son's medication trial has begun?

By learning everything you can about the disorder(s) your child has, the accepted treatments, and specifically the medications used, you can be an active collaborator in your child's treatment rather than a passive and helpless bystander. Additional information on the medications can be obtained not only from this book and your child's doctor but also from your pharmacist, libraries, and the many parent-run support groups on the different child disorders.

Lots of supportive measures can also be helpful with children who have psychiatric disorders. Consistency in parenting and firm but understanding discipline can minimize your child's daily stress. Over the long haul, focus less on specifics such as grades and more on instilling *love and confidence* in your child while ensuring that the child is acquiring an acceptable fund of knowledge. You might also consider parent training for a difficult child. Practice child advocacy with the other adults in your child's life—your child should know that you are always in his corner. Don't forget to take care of yourself while you're taking care of your child: Get involved in "respite" programs, where your child spends a day or a weekend with another family and you return the favor at another time, or get away yourselves for periodic evenings and weekends. And at all times, do whatever you can to keep your sense of humor!

You should also keep a detailed record of your child's treatment history, including a separate page that lists medication trials. Many doctors keep on hand a similar summary of the child's problems as well as the different medications used for the child's treatment (in addition to the more detailed records in the child's file). I, for one, find it very helpful to have this to refer to when I have been treating a child with different medications over several years. I encourage parents to keep a three-ring notebook of their child's treatment history that includes copies of all testing and evaluations. I also advocate using a medication log, such as the one on page 115, containing information on each medication tried: when, at what dose, and what happened—whether it worked as expected and whether it produced any side effects. See pages 270–271 in the Appendix for a sample medication log and a blank log for you to photocopy and use as needed.

Parents who keep such logs are not at the mercy of a clinic's medical records when they need information on their child's treatment history. This is particularly important today, when employers keep changing their group health insurance plans and when groups are often subjected to the managed care that shunts patients from office to office and doctor to doctor. Parents who have their child's treatment histories at their fingertips simply have an edge.

You can give your child's doctor an edge, too, by expressing your openness to having other practitioners get involved in your child's case

TABLE 4. Example of a Medication Log for a Child Treated for ADHD

Start date	Medication	Daily dose	Response	Side effect(s)
1/03	Ritalin	40 mg SR	OK	Poor appetite, weight loss
9/03	Dexedrine	30 mg	Good	Nervousness, picking
1/04	Clonidine	0.3 mg	None	Sedation
3/04	Strattera	50 mg	Good	Dry mouth, ± improved attention
5/04	Strattera + Adderall XR	50 mg 10 mg (Adderall XR)	Very good	Dry mouth

whenever a sticky question or issue arises. Recently one of my colleagues consulted me when he found no drug besides very-high-dose imipramine helpful for his patient's ADHD and depression. Together we were able to arrive at adding low-dose Effexor to the child's medication regimen, which allowed the doctor to lower the dose of imipramine. Some parents request that physicians contact other doctors and offer to pay for additional supervision or formal consultation on the case, such as telephone contacts.

You also might find yourself becoming a sort of "team coordinator" for your child's health care providers. If, for instance, your child is receiving individual psychotherapy by someone other than the prescribing practitioner, you will want to ensure that the care is adequately coordinated. Since the individual therapist is generally seeing the child more often than the practitioner responsible for monitoring the medication, it is helpful for the therapist to relay by verbal or written communication his or her impressions of the child, family, and other systems relevant to the child's care (school, afterschool programs, groups). You should sign releases allowing bidirectional communication between or among these caregivers. You, too, should be kept updated on your child's progress, or lack thereof, in therapy. In turn, the therapist can help by working with you in following the progress of a medication trial.

Now that your role as captain of your child's treatment team has become more and more important, keep in mind that throughout your child's care you'll be handling multiple tasks, from getting any educational ac-commodations that your child needs from the school to working with your insurance company or the state's insurance program for children to en-sure that your child is eligible for a broad variety of evaluation and treat-ment programs for the children by competent clinicians. Meanwhile, you have to oversee that the psychotherapy and medication management are being completed properly and that the medications ordered and filled at the pharmacy are correct and that the child takes them at the correct times.

Finally, the most important job you have is to monitor your child's progress. You are in a position to see the child in his normal surround-ings, and you can observe day-by-day changes. You are the indispens-able eyes and ears of the professional caregivers. Please don't fall prey to analyzing your child's progress and side effects minute by minute, though. We've found this practice is deleterious to the child's and family's adaptation to the disorder and daily functioning because such "micromanagement" often causes parents to stop seeing the forest for the trees.

Do I have to change anything in my daughter's daily routine to make sure she gets the full effect of her medication?

This is a question for the prescriber, because it depends on the prescrip-tion, the disorder, and other factors in your daughter's unique situation. An infinite number of factors might interfere with metabolism of the drug, but the major offenders that my colleagues and I have observed are other medications, herbal remedies, special diet supplements, and exposure to toxins (sniffing gasoline and working around organic cleaners, mainly tolu-ene-based). When the medication trial begins, inform the doctor about any of these that are part of your daughter's environment and ask what to do about them as well as any other potential interference.

Will my son need to change his diet?

The vast majority of psychotropic medications do not require any specific diet. The rare exception are the monoamine oxidase inhibitors (MAOIs), Parnate and Nardil, which require a strict diet but are not commonly pre-scribed for children. Your child's doctor or the pharmacist will be able to provide an extensive list of foods and medications that should be avoided if this family of medications is prescribed for your child.

Is it OK to use OTC drugs at the same time as the prescription?

Most OTC medications in pediatric groups can be used safely with the medications described in this book. However, it is always prudent to discuss this with your pharmacist and/or doctor. The majority of potential interactions are more minor and include the child being overly sedated, as is the case for the standard antihistamines, or mildly agitated, as with the decongestants. When in doubt, for a cold or allergies, Benadryl (diphenhydramine), ChlorTrimeton (chlorpheniramine), or similar medications are generally safe and effective. Most medicines for stomachaches or headaches do not interact with the medications your child will be taking; however, Tagamet, Pepcid, and Axid may increase blood levels of certain medicines. If your child is receiving one of the antidepressants—Prozac, Paxil, Zoloft, Luvox, Effexor, or Serzone—you should contact your doctor if you plan to use one of the new types of less sedative seasonal allergy medications such as Tavist or Hismanal. Because of potential drug interactions with these medications, Claritin, Zyrtec, and Allegra are the suggested antihistamines. Children receiving an infrequently used class of antidepressants called *monoamine oxidase inhibitors* need to adhere closely not only to their special diet but also to prohibitions against taking over-the-counter medications without consulting their pharmacist and doctor.

> **antihistamines:** A class of medications that block histamine receptors or histamine release. Used primarily to treat allergies, they are used commonly in psychiatry to treat drug reactions and for their sedative properties.

What about other prescriptions?

Since you've undoubtedly stayed up all night with a sick child at some time in the past, it would be frivolous to remind you that children occasionally have medical problems necessitating other medications. When that happens, it is important to notify the person examining your child of the current agent your child is taking even if he has missed a dose earlier. In general, most of the antibiotics are safe and well tolerated with the psychotropic medications. Doses of codeine or other narcotic pain medications (Percodan) can often be reduced because your child's current psychotropic medications make them work better. Likewise, you can often give less of the prescribed cough medicines when your child is receiving psychoactive medications. Medicines for heartburn or ulcers should be administered at times other than those when your child is receiving the medications for emotional and behavioral disorders.

Emphasize to your child how important it is to resist taking illicit drugs, including marijuana. Explain that we just don't understand all the potential drug interactions, and they could be very dangerous. Alcohol should also be avoided, since people who drink while on psychotropic medications report getting drunk faster, feeling nauseated, and having a severe hangover even when drinking in moderation.

Can I substitute generics for brand names?

As you probably know, the brand name—Ritalin, for example—is the name chosen carefully for the specific medication by the pharmaceutical company that developed that medication. The generic name—such as methylphenidate—is the medication's chemical name. In this book and in general, brand names are capitalized, whereas generics are not. Brand name medication is generally more expensive than the generic, whether you pay directly or you have a copay insurance policy.

It is the brand name product that has been studied extensively by the pharmaceutical company under guidelines and monitoring by the FDA. Both the pharmacological properties of the medication and the "vehicle" (specific capsule, pill, or tablet) that the medication is put in to keep it stable and palatable for humans have been evaluated. There is also a quality control from batch to batch of medication, which generally ensures that each tablet of the medication from month to month is virtually identical in the amount of medication and filler it contains. Generic versions do not undergo the same rigor in development. In addition, a number of pharmaceutical companies make generic versions of medications, so pharmacies often sell different versions of the same medication from month to month based on the cost to them. Of note is the fact that pharmacies often profit more from selling you the generic version than the brand name medication, despite the price differential to you or your insurance company.

Most generic medications are well manufactured and have pharmacological properties that make them acceptable, less expensive alternatives to the brand name medication. On an individual basis, some parents report no difference between the brand and generic preparations, whereas others note loss of effectiveness, allergic reactions, or more side effects with the generic versions. Reports in the medical literature claim that marked differences may exist; in particular, the anticonvulsants are said to be inferior, carrying a notably higher risk for seizures. Specifically, for example, Tegretol, the branded drug, is advisable over the generic, carbamazepine.

I advise using the brand name medicine when starting treatment and then trying the generic only if your child has had a good response to treatment. With this approach, you avoid the treatment failure or side effects that sometimes result from using a poor generic drug. There are, however, no absolute guidelines for deciding between generics and brand names, and many parents have taken the approach of trying a small prescription of a generic and then continuing with it if it proves to be well tolerated and effective.

Be sure to discuss your concerns about different producers of the generic forms of the medication with the pharmacist. Knowing which pharmaceutical company is making the generic your child is taking can facilitate consistency in the way your child's body interacts with the medication. Common and well-respected companies that specialize in generic psychotropic compounds include Geneva, Zenith, and Burr. Some generic preparations of medications may also be made by other major pharmaceutical companies, such as the commonly prescribed generic version of nortriptyline, which is also sold under the trade name Aventyl. If your child has been on a stable regimen and doing relatively well and develops a drug reaction, or loses the response to the medication, first check to see if the recent batch of medication was a different version of the medication or if the pharmacist received other reports of problems with the medicine. Although infrequent, I have a number of parents who have noted loss of effectiveness related to a particular "batch" of medicine.

COLLABORATION EQUALS SAFETY

If your child is experiencing severe psychiatric symptoms or is abusing substances, you'll have to be especially vigilant and diligent in your communications with the child's therapist and physician. The child's therapist should brief you if your child develops active suicidality, hallucinations, or substance abuse, or becomes a danger to herself or to others. Should the child require psychiatric hospitalization or substance abuse treatment, your therapist should work in concert with the prescribing practitioner. Your child's therapist should also be very involved in working with the various systems with which your child is involved, particularly school.

I feel like I'm constantly hovering over my child as it is. What more do
I have to do to monitor this medication trial?

Monitoring doesn't have to mean hovering. You'll probably find, in fact,
that once you settle into a routine, you no longer feel the nervous need to
check on your child constantly.

By closely observing and reporting on your child's reaction to the
medication, you will be collaborating with treatment, and this in turn will
lessen your own sense of helplessness regarding your child's problem.

Your ongoing surveillance system should include attention to administration of the drug(s), the child's adherence with the treatment plan, the
effectiveness of the treatment, and its side effects. As you can imagine,
your medication log (see page 115) can play a useful role in keeping track.
First, though, you need to devise a system:

1. To improve your child's likelihood of taking the medication on
time and in the proper quantity, work out a routine system of medication administration. Whether you tie in the administration with
an event (mealtime) or the time on the clock, make sure it's easy
for your child to make it part of his daily routine.

2. Adherence is crucial to the effectiveness of your child's treatment,
so you will have to plan to talk to and observe your child to ensure
he is actually taking the medication. One of the major reasons for
medication failure in adolescents is simply nonadherence.

3. If you receive feedback from your child and family, you can gather
a lot of information about the medication's effectiveness and side
effects without hovering over the child. Be sure to ask your child
and family about these concerns periodically.

> **adherence**: Following the guidelines agreed on by you
> and the provider, including taking medication as
> prescribed.

A major goal in any medication trial is to establish the optimum dosage for your child. Your reporting based on close observation of your child
can give the doctor an idea of whether the dose is too low to have a positive effect, too high to avoid undesirable side effects, or somewhere in between. Although generally only a nuisance, side effects may signal more
dangerous problems with a medication such as a drug reaction. Likewise,
more subtle side effects such as indigestion may adversely affect your

child's compliance. Discovering side effects may not only improve safety and compliance but also help the doctor arrive at the right dosage more quickly than without your input.

Because we all make mistakes, at the beginning of the trial, your child's doctor should also describe the signs that you've given too much medication to your child. Children who are receiving too much stimulant, for example, may stare, pick at their skin, or report an uneasy feeling.

How can I monitor a medication trial when my child spends most of his day at school?

With the use of extended-release medications (for ADHD), parents can observe the child's behavior long after the school day ends. In addition, you can monitor medication effectiveness during the weekends, afternoons, evenings, and mornings. The school should be able to give you frequent updates on your child's progress if the state's privacy laws allow, possibly using behavior rating scales. The child's school performance itself, in fact, is a way of measuring the effectiveness of the medication. Follow the suggestions on pages 109–112 for communicating with a designated school advocate and the nurse.

How do we tell if the drug is working?

First, try to be open-minded and objective while you watch for positive effects (or side effects). Sometimes parents can end up biased by the doctor's hopes and expectations. Ask the doctor for precise signs of response in target symptoms (the major problems being treated) as well as a time frame in which they should appear.

Determining effectiveness of an agent is easier if your child's behavior occurs all the time, as with hyperactivity or anxiety, and thus responds more dramatically. Behaviors such as intermittent outbursts or infrequent panic attacks are more difficult to assess and are best described by how often and severe they are when they occur. The signs that a drug is working may include improvement in sleep, energy level, socialization, and mood for depressed children. Anxious children, in addition to feeling less nervous, should have fewer stomachaches. Youth with bipolar disorder will have fewer outbursts and less irritability. Obsessional children will not spend as much time with rituals or their obsessions. Children with ADHD will have improved attention, less impulsivity, and less hyperactivity. These are very general examples. If you and your child's practitioner have

developed a solid understanding of your child's problem, together you will
be able to come up with signs to watch for in your particular child: If
Tommy usually retreats to his room after school when depressed, talking
to you or going out to play when he gets home may be a sign that his medication is working. If Tanya's biggest ADHD challenge is concentrating on
homework, finishing a 15-minute assignment on her own may be a major
milestone.

Very roughly, it usually takes at least 1 month to determine if a medication is working, leading many physicians to request a routine follow-up
visit in 4 weeks. Monthly to bimonthly visits are typical during the first
few months of treatment. During these visits, your doctor will be assessing the effectiveness of the medication, any side effects, and whether your
child is taking the medication. Once the regimen is working and your
child's condition is improving or stable, the interval between visits may be
widened to 3, 4, or even 6 months. Children with certain conditions such
as mood disorders often require frequent visits for a prolonged period of
time.

As a parent, you should be satisfied that your child (and family) is
benefiting from a medication. You should see proof of efficacy in your deal-
ings with the child and get objective information from the school. Don't be
surprised if your view or the school's differs from your child's view. Some
kids are simply poor reporters of their own illness and response to medications. It is not uncommon for me to have a child or adolescent report no
difference in behavior while the school and family state that the medication is working very well. Such may be the case in ADHD and bipolar disorder—yet, of interest, kids with anxiety disorders or depression often
are more accurate reporters of their progress.

What types of side effects should I watch for?

Parents and children should expect side effects; no medication comes
without them. While it is important that you ask your children about side
effects, try not to amplify problems that were probably there prior to use
of the medication, such as insomnia. The careful observation of your child
that a medication trial calls for may subject you to overreading physical or
behavioral signs as side effects when they were actually present before
the medication was started. This "amplification phenomenon" led the
mother of 14-year-old Don to report to me that the Ativan I had prescribed
for his anxiety was causing temper tantrums. Don's psychiatric problems
also included severe behavioral outbursts, and when his mother and I re-

viewed the number and types of tantrums he had been having after a week on the medication, we could see that they were no different than before the medication; it was just that Don's mother was now more attentive to his state. Similarly, studies with stimulants show that the majority of side effects reported while children were taking stimulants predated the administration of the stimulants.

I suggest asking the pharmacist for a readable printout of the side effects and how to use the medication. Most pharmacies also carry detailed package inserts that give detailed information found in the *PDR* on each medication.

Talk to anyone whose child is taking a psychotropic medication and you will undoubtedly hear horror stories about side effects. Without a doubt, side effects remain among the most problematic aspects of using medicines in anybody, particularly children. But since all medications have them, you might as well be familiar with the same general principles that doctors use in working with and managing side effects.

The majority of side effects can be anticipated based on the known properties of the drug. For example, children receiving clonidine or Valium for anxiety problems often complain, at least initially, of being tired, which is technically referred to as *somnolence* or *lethargy*. Some of the newer antidepressants such as Prozac or Zoloft cause upset stomachs or headaches. Trazodone, imipramine, and other older antidepressants often cause dry mouth and constipation. Children receiving Adderall and other stimulant-class agents often have a lowered appetite, whereas those taking antipsychotics such as Risperdal or Zyprexa have an increased appetite. Children on lithium urinate and drink fluids more frequently.

Other side effects, generally less frequent, are unexpected (*idiosyncratic*) and are difficult to anticipate. For example, unanticipated rashes, blood problems, and worsening of the underlying condition may occur during medication treatment. Seizures may also occur and may even signal an underlying yet undetected problem. The following are the more common side effects noted in my practice.

Sedation. Sedation (sleepiness) is a frequent side effect that often gets less severe with time. Be sure to determine whether the sedation is occurring 1–3 hours after the agent is given or during the wearoff of the compound. Sedation occurring soon after the medication is given is probably related directly to the compound. This is the case for clonidine, the antipsychotic medications like Trilafon or Seroquel, and the Valium-like benzodiazepines. If a medicine causes your child to become tired, consider giving the medication before sleep. In that way, the sedation caused by the agent occurs during sleep. As mentioned, sedating agents can be your ally if your child is having difficulty with sleep. Sedation occurring many hours after the medication is given is probably related to a wearoff or "crash" from the medication. Dexedrine tablets and other short-acting stimulant medications are notorious for causing this. Often, changing to an extended-release preparation of the agent or giving a small repeat dose of the medication eliminates the crash.

Rashes. A common unpredictable side effect is a rash that often starts 2–6 weeks after the new use of the responsible agent. Generally, the rash associated with the psychotropics is more a discomfort but not life-threatening, as are some of the rashes related to the antibiotics. These rashes are generally red, occur more on the trunk of the child, and itch (are *pruritic*). The presence of this type of rash may not mean that your child will have to be taken off the medication. A severe rash with involvement of the inside of the mouth or in the palms of the hands or feet in children should be reported immediately. This may represent an infrequent condition reported in those receiving Tegretol or Lamictal. There is a higher likelihood of having another rash with a different medication within the same family of medication. For example, children on desipramine may also have a rash on nortriptyline. Your child's practitioner may choose to continue the medication if the rash is not severe, with careful monitoring. Often, Benadryl is used to counteract the itching and discomfort associated with a rash and is safely coadministered with most psychotropics.

The opposite reaction. Another very disconcerting side effect of psychotropics, particularly in children who are being treated for outbursts or hyperactivity, is the worsening of the problem with the medication (*paradoxical response*). A small group of children, for example, may not become less anxious or less agitated with a minor tranquilizer such as Valium or Klonopin but will, instead, become more nervous or have severe agitation *as a side effect* (generally referred to as *disinhibition*). These children may act silly, giddy, or even manic. Some children will become more depressed on the antidepressants. Children receiving lithium for mood problems may get more agitated and moody. Children may become more hyperactive on the stimulants and be unable to sleep on the sleep-aiding medications. Seven-year-old Troy had a severe anxiety problem characterized by nervousness, inability to separate, and social inhibition. After two single doses of Ambien, Troy was touching other kids, laughing inappropriately, talking excessively, and goofing around—all entirely out of character. After 2 hours, this disinhibition reaction diminished, and Troy is now doing well on Buspar. Recent data suggest that if your child has a "paradoxical effect" from one medicine, he or she will have a 50% chance of another such reaction to another medication in the same family.

Somatic reactions. Other side effects may not be observable by you or your child but occur within the body and affect the blood or internal organs. For this reason, your child may require medical monitoring. The most commonly employed tests for the psychotropics are the EKG and blood tests. The EKG is often completed before starting your child on medication, again during the initiation of a medication trial, and less frequently thereafter. Since some of the medications, such as imipramine and desipramine, may subtly alter the electrical system of the heart, an EKG is used to ensure that these changes are not severe. Other medications may influence red and white blood cell production. Such examples include Tegretol affecting white blood cell counts and Clozaril affecting red and white blood cells. For Tegretol, periodic monitoring of white blood cell counts is advisable, and for Clozaril, weekly to biweekly complete blood counts (red and white) are required. Blood tests are also necessary for monitoring to ensure that your child's kidneys are handling certain medications such as lithium and Neurontin. Children receiving Cylert and Depakote will need periodic basic blood tests to ensure that there are no adverse effects on their liver. Similarly, your child's thyroid tests should be checked occasionally if she is on lithium.

---

somatic: Referring to the body, as opposed to the mind.

What should I do if I do notice a side effect in my child?

If you can do so (ask your doctor if you're not sure), take measures to counteract the side effect, such as administering sedating medications at night instead of in the morning. If the side effects are interfering with the child's functioning or school performance, call the doctor. Every doctor has a different approach here, so discuss with the practitioner how to contact him or her for routine and emergency situations. It is also a good idea to have a contingency plan for when you cannot get in touch with the doctor. On more than one occasion, I have had the battery in my beeper stop working without my realizing it! You should have another plan for times when your child ends up at risk or is a danger to anyone else—options such as using a mental health crisis center, emergency room, or in the case of severe behavioral outbursts, involvement of the local police should be discussed with your child's doctor.

For the vast majority of problems, routine messages left with the office receptionist or on the doctor's voice mail or e-mail are adequate. Leave the times and numbers where you can be reached. You'll find voice mail or an answering machine of your own helpful for getting uncomplicated answers when you're not available to receive the doctor's return call. In more urgent situations, page your child's doctor immediately. If you are requesting an immediate callback, try to keep the phone line clear and provide the doctor with basic information on your child. If you should reach the physician covering for your doctor, give a very brief history of your child: "Dr. Spencer treats my son, who is a 14-year-old with bipolar disorder who is currently telling me that he is hearing loud voices in his head. Dr. Spencer started him on Zoloft 2 weeks ago because he was depressed and was concerned that he might get agitated and asked me to call him immediately if this occurred." By relaying this amount of information as efficiently as she did, this mother enabled me to make changes over the phone and avert more serious problems. In this case, the child's hallucinations disappeared 1 day after stopping the Zoloft. I also asked the mother to update me the next day, which she did by leaving a message on my voice mail.

I ask the parents of my patients to call my office if a side effect appears that has not been described by me and is worrisome to the parent. For example, rashes, headaches, motor tics, nausea, and sleep disturbance should be called in to your doctor. Since not all problems will be related to the medication, a brief discussion will help detect how the medicine and the side effect are related. If the problem turns out to be related to the medication, your doctor may have suggestions for eliminating the side effect and making your child feel more comfortable. For example, children who develop nausea on medications may benefit from taking the medication with a meal.

Any severe side effects such as shortness of breath, chest discomfort, severe agitation, fainting, or disorientation call for immediate contact with your child's doctor even if they are occurring infrequently.

You should feel comfortable calling (or, less frequently, paging) your doctor for advice on what may be happening or what to do to remedy a course. Paging your doctor may be necessary if there is a paradoxical response to the medication (e.g., your child has panic attacks on a medicine for anxiety), a serious side effect, or reason to fear that your child is going to harm himself or others. Remember, this is a limited experience for you, but your doctor has a number of cases and a broader experience in dealing with medication problems.

I don't think this medication is working, but my doctor wants us to stick with it. How do I know if he's right?

It helps to limit your expectations of medication trials and to anticipate "bumps" along the way. Your child's doctor does not have a crystal ball and will not be able to foretell which medicine will be most effective and tolerable for your child. Therefore, you and your child need to be ready to try different agents with the understanding that there will most probably be successes and failures along the medication journey. The keys are persistence and systematic trials of different agents within and between classes of medication.

In the case of Gene, an 11-year-old I treat for anxiety and ADHD, the stimulants Ritalin and Cylert had little effect on the ADHD and made his anxiety worse. Desipramine made him feel terrible, and Effexor helped the anxiety at the expense of nausea. Wellbutrin was helpful for aspects of his ADHD but had little effect on his anxiety, and he disinhibited (became giddy) when I added Valium to the Wellbutrin to treat the anxiety. Buspar did nothing for the anxiety. Finally, after he was placed on nortriptyline, there was a meaningful diminution in anxiety and, to a lesser degree, ADHD. Dexedrine was added for further ADHD coverage. Both Gene and his mother were patient through this protracted series of trials, which spanned 5 months, and now Gene is doing much better because of their perseverance.

Even in the face of a medication trial failure, you need to have the attitude that it is worth hanging in there to continue finding out what may be helpful for your child. It is also important to be sure that you have a doctor who has the same philosophy.

We've already tried three drugs, and they've had awful side effects and little positive result. Isn't it time to try something besides medication?

If after multiple trials there is still no response, a careful review of the situation is warranted. First, make sure you and the doctor still agree with the original diagnostic hypothesis. If the child's symptoms seem to have changed, or new ones have appeared, you may want to reevaluate the child. Next, go over possible contributing stressors, your child's adherence to the medication regime, and any medical conditions that may be interfering with treatment.

A thorough review of past trials and outcomes is also in order. By keeping a log of medication trials including maximum doses, outcome, and major side effects, you can work with your child's doctor in determining classes (such as stimulants) and specific agents (Klonopin vs. Ativan) that have not been considered. Don't be shy about suggesting different agents that may not have been tried. More than once, parents have wanted me to try a specific agent on their child because of a friend's child's response to the agent, and although the chosen agent may not have been my logical next choice, the child has responded nicely.

Sometimes, on the other hand, a break from a medication trial is advised. If the child has had to suffer debilitating side effects such as a painful rash or disturbing panic attacks, both the child and the parents may be understandably hesitant to keep trying. Unfortunately, we still rely on trial and error in finding the correct psychotropic drug for young people. The best move, then, may be to take a break until the child and parents can regain their confidence in medication trials.

We've gotten along fine with this doctor so far, but now that we can't seem to find the right medications, everyone is getting very testy. Should we start looking for a new doctor?

The relationship between you and your child's doctor is often tested during both a crisis and ongoing unsuccessful medication trials. Obviously it is important to have good communication with your child's treater through this process. As with most of life, keeping your sense of humor while sharing your frustration over the situation with your child's doctor can be useful to maintaining your own mental health and keeping communication lines open.

Although you may feel angry, exasperated, and helpless about the situation, try not to blame the doctor if your child is not responding to treatment—as long as the doctor has been working with you and has been competently and systematically trying reasonable agents for your child. Being the mortal beings that we are, doctors are vulnerable to the same emotions and disappointments as patients and their families. I try to see children who are not responding to treatment as a challenge, yet on certain days it can seem more like a burden. Sometimes without realizing what is occurring, doctors may blame their patients or their families for the child's doing poorly. Doctors may also unconsciously become unresponsive to the needs of a patient or simply make themselves unavailable. For a discussion of when to get a second opinion, see page 83.

I saw 8-year-old Robert after his treating pediatrician had a "frank" discussion with Robert's parents in which he told them they were responsible for his poor response to the traditional ADHD medication because they were not taking the situation seriously. Apparently they were in the habit of joking about his impulsivity and talking openly about his spaciness: "Just like his Aunt May." He in turn would joke that he really was quite smart but that knowing everybody's business in class would make him a better principal when he grew up. In fact, everyone in this family was very committed to treatment but was exercising the very healthy defense of humor. They knew of the ongoing ADHD problems, but rather than damaging Robert's self-esteem (or letting him berate himself), they brought up the problematic symptoms in a less direct manner. In this case, the more pressing problem was with the doctor, who felt frustrated, angry, and injured because the young man did not respond to treatment. Robert did eventually respond fairly well to a combination of antihypertensives, antidepressants . . . and humor.

> **antihypertensives:** A class of medications used to reduce blood pressure; also found to be useful for certain psychiatric disorders, such as ADHD or Tourette's syndrome.

If you notice this type of attitude in your child's doctor, discuss it if at all possible. Voicing your commitment to working with your child's doctor as a team, toward whatever treatment will help the child, may give your collaboration the boost it needs. You can also do your part as a team player by being sure to keep appointments and acknowledge the frustration and hopelessness that both of you feel during these medication trials.

Certainly, however, if you are dissatisfied with the level of care provided by your child's practitioner, you should seek an alternative view of the care being provided. An increasing number of parents of children who are receiving care in an HMO or under tightly controlled managed care have also sought outside consultation to ensure that the care is in the child's best interest and not necessarily that of the corporation managing the care. Besides seeking a second physician's opinion, you might ask for insight from other professionals such as therapists working with your child who have knowledge of and experience with medications.

Consultations for children not responding to treatment should be focused and include a medication review, educational review, assessment of the family system, and a psychological profile. To optimize the process, I suggest writing down specific questions you would like to have addressed during the consultation. Areas that you may want to ask more about include what is wrong, what is the typical course of your child's disorder, what treatments are most effective, what are the next two or three pharmacological trials the consultant would consider, and when the prescriber would suggest a follow-up visit if your child is still having difficulty.

It took us a year and four different drugs to arrive at a drug regimen that worked, and for 2 years everything has been pretty good. Now my son's symptoms are returning even though he's still taking the drug. Why?

The most common causes of loss of effect are tolerance to the medication and the need for an increase in dosage because of the child's growth. Other reasons for the sudden loss of effect include nonadherence, co-administration of another drug that may be interacting, environmental stressors such as parental separation, a bad batch of the medication, or the conversion to a generic compound.

Although there are no clearcut reasons why children stop responding to their medication, there are three major speculations on what may be occurring: (1) that the brain may be adapting to the medication with subtle changes in the nerve-to-nerve communication; (2) that the amount of medication actually reaching the brain may be changing; or (3) that another disorder may have emerged in the child.

Increasingly active symptoms of the child's disorder should always sound a warning bell. Sometimes the underlying disorder is being treated aggressively enough, but the child begins to act out socially, perform poorly academically, or express displeasure that doesn't seem to pass. In that case, you might have to consider a change in the environment (such as the school) or the addition of other therapies such as individual psychotherapy, group psychotherapy, a big-brother program, a camp, or another resource. Your child's doctor should be able to lead you to appropriate sources.

My son has been on medication for a year now, and he's doing so well I'm beginning to wonder if he needs his pills anymore. Should I try taking him off the drugs?

It's not a good idea to stop giving a child his medication without talking to the doctor first. Some drugs need to be tapered off slowly (see the pertinent chapter in Part III), but it is also possible that your child's doctor will disagree with trying to wean him off the medication right now. Psychotropic drugs do not cure psychiatric or psychological disorders. On the other hand, some conditions do prove to be "self-righting" in some children, which is one reason to reassess the need for pharmacotherapy by tapering and discontinuing the medications periodically. This taper should be considered if your child is free of symptoms for a significant period of time, which should be the doctor's call. After 14-year-old Maria had been treated successfully for depression with 20 mg of Celexa daily for 1½ years, we decided to try tapering off her medication. First we reduced her dosage to 10 mg daily and watched her closely for the next 2 months. Then we administered 10 mg every other day and again observed her for 2 months. When her symptoms did not reappear, we discontinued the Celexa altogether. At her 2-year follow-up, Maria is doing very well.

> **self-righting**: Returning to normal functioning on one's own.

Unfortunately, in the majority of psychiatric disturbances, the effectiveness of the medications is seen only when they are being taken, with little lasting effectiveness if they are discontinued.

Everyone can see that our daughter's condition has improved with this new treatment, but for some reason she takes every opportunity to skip a dose. Why?

Dr. Ross Baldessarini, a professor of psychiatry at Harvard Medical School, teaches that the most important impediment to a medication's getting into the bloodstream is the patient's not taking the medication. For a variety of reasons, children and adolescents will refuse to take medications. Among the more common causes in younger children are side effects. Typically, young children will not alert their parents to their headaches or stomachaches but, instead, refuse to take the medicine. Children may not like the taste of the medicine or may complain that the medicine is getting caught in their throat—a very uncomfortable feeling! In that case, you can have your child practice swallowing with something non-threatening like tiny breath mint candies. Speaking to the pharmacist about different formulations (sprinkles or chewable formulations) and methods of taking the medication (such as opening capsules) may help eliminate many of these problems. New forms of some medications make it easier for kids to take their medicine; you'll find more information on these in Parts II and III. If getting your child the medication she needs means mixing it with applesauce, and the pharmacist says that's OK, just do it—insisting on her swallowing a pill is not worth the battle. Be careful that you talk with someone knowledgeable prior to changing how your child takes her medication, though. Children should not, for example, chew extended-release tablets.

Children often report stopping medications because they "felt different," so before you assume side effects, try to determine if your child is describing only the predicted effects of the medication.

Some children stop taking their medications because they are embarrassed by taking medications, particularly in school. Initiating a discussion with your child about the reason for taking the medication may help. But you can also ask the child's doctor about long-acting preparations—Dexedrine spansules instead of tablets, for example—to eliminate the need to administer medication during the school day.

Other young people are afraid of the consequences of taking any medications. Often they need direction in distinguishing prescribed medication from illicit substances. In these instances, directly addressing the child's concern and reducing side effects often alleviate adherence issues.

My teenager avoids taking his medicine because he says it just keeps reminding him that he's not "normal." How can I help him with this?

Just like adults, children and adolescents worry about whether their bodies and minds are OK. It is important for them to understand that they have treatable problems that were not brought on by themselves, are not products of sin or signs of moral weakness, do not indicate intellectual deficits (generally), and are simply not their fault. Medications can help reset the brain chemistry and help in eliminating or managing these problems.

If you can get these facts across to your child, terrific. But you may need help, and you shouldn't be afraid to ask for it. Resistance to taking medication is a very common therapeutic issue, and it should be addressed by your child's practitioner. Often it's a matter of control; your child may view you as "forcing" him to take medication, which means any explanation that comes from you won't have much persuasive power. If your son has ever given you the idea that he believes he has to take medication because in your eyes he is "sick" or "crazy," consult the prescriber or a therapist.

Sometimes, in concert with the adolescent, I agree to a taper in the medication, even if it appears to be premature, with the understanding that we *all* agree to restart the medicine if the teenager has a return of the problem.

If the problem is that the child feels ashamed of having a disorder, you can help by pointing out examples of the many others who have the same problems—either friends and relatives that you know about or, even better sometimes, famous adults who are leading successful lives with the same disorder. Websites dedicated to your child's disorder as well as books on the disorder aimed at parents often contain these names.

Should my teenager or I be responsible for her medication?

As your child's parent or guardian, you will need to assume responsibility for the medication until your child is 18 years old. That is not to say that you can't share some of this responsibility with your child as she gets older, but the bottom line remains that you are responsible for her well-being. You are the keeper of the medicine and should dispense daily doses to your child.

Because many of the medicines can be fatal in overdose, you should keep them safely away from siblings who may inadvertently mistake the colorful pills and tablets for candy. Unfortunately, many overdoses and deaths on medications occur not in the patient but in a sibling—who has taken the medication either accidentally or in a suicide attempt. Children also often get into their parents' medications. For children at risk of misusing their agents, such as substance abusers or suicidal children, the medication needs to be stowed and inventoried carefully. Medications with abuse potential such as the Valium-like medications (benzodiazepines) or the stimulants should be administered carefully and kept in a safe place (avoid medicine cabinets). Some parents have a locking drawer or cabinet in which they store their children's medication. Of interest, it is generally not the child for whom the medication is prescribed who abuses the compounds but the child's friends or friends of a friend. Even then, a recent survey indicates that less than 1% of high school seniors have tried Ritalin, Adderall, or like compounds that were not prescribed for them, and in the majority of cases, this was only once and by mouth. As with most medications, there is potential for abuse of the stimulants; this potential appears to be the least with Cylert, intermediate with Ritalin, and the most with Desoxyn (methamphetamine). The extended-release stimulants have the lowest abuse potential.

I'm worried about having my son's stimulants around the house. What is the best way to keep everyone safe from any kind of misuse?

The number-one safety measure, as just discussed, is to supervise all of the psychotropics being administered to your child, whatever the child's age. Whenever medications are available, there is legitimate reason for concern about overdose. This means that proper storage is just as important as parental supervision. All medication should be inaccessible to anyone but the parents, preferably locked away in a separate cabinet. Compounds such as the tricyclic antidepressants (desipramine, imipramine, and others), lithium, Tegretol, Depakote, and clonidine can be very dangerous in overdose. Old or ineffective psychotropics should be disposed of immediately.

As I've mentioned before, many overdoses are accidental and befall someone other than the person for whom the prescription is written. However, if your child is depressed and at risk for misusing the medication, talk to the doctor about using weekly prescriptions and prescribing medications with less lethality in overdose (such as Prozac, Zoloft, Luvox, Celexa, Lexapro, and Wellbutrin).

Besides actually taking the medication, what should my child's role be in the course of drug treatment?

Children should be encouraged to be involved in their treatment from the diagnostic evaluation through adherence with the prescribed regimen and monitoring of the drugs' effects on them. They should also be taught to recognize and report side effects.

Despite their disorder, children also need to be encouraged to work hard at mastering their academic, social, interpersonal, and behavioral skills. I joke to my patients that I have never seen a Ritalin tablet jump up on a desk and do a child's homework for her. It's very important not to simply attribute improvements in symptoms to the medication itself. Help family members and school staff avoid statements such as "You're doing so well this past week, you must be taking your medication!" Rather, emphasize that medicine is one part of the overall treatment plan and that you know your child is trying hard to do his or her best. The medicine simply helps the child be the best he or she can be.

As children become adolescents, they will (and should) have more say in their medications. To enhance adherence, be sure that your adolescent is talking with the prescriber about his or her condition and the positive and negative effects of the medication. Often the adolescent will request a trial off medication to see if in fact the medicine is needed. In general, this can be managed by agreeing to taper the medication but to restart it if symptoms reappear. When carefully executed, I have found this invaluable to engage the teenager in the responsible care of his or her own condition.

What is a medication holiday?

A medication holiday is a period of time (usually 1–3 months) during which the child's medication is discontinued. Medication holidays are commonly used over the summer months for ADHD that predominately affects a child's academic performance or for anxiety in which the child's major stress occurs during the academic year. Medication holidays are used to reduce the total load of medication and are thought to help children "catch up" on problems that presumably result from medication usage. For example, many children are taken off their Ritalin over the summer to enhance their appetite and help them catch up on their weight. Medication holidays are not appropriate for the bulk of children and adolescents who suffer from illness that is pervasive and causes social or family difficulties.

WHEN CHILDREN NEED TO BE HOSPITALIZED

A few of the children who are being treated with medications, by the nature of their underlying problem, may still need hospitalization. It is important to note that the hospitalization is often secondary to the severity of the problem and the inability of the medication to contain the condition. This development naturally causes anxiety in parents, and they often have many questions about when, why, and how children need to be hospitalized. Because children are being sent out of hospitals much faster now (the typical length of stay is 1 week), parents and families are having to deal with sicker kids, and the outpatient system (including counselors and schools) is having to manage these youth while they are still quite unstable.

Commensurate with reduced hospitalization, there has been an increase in the utilization of day treatment facilities (caring for the child during the day in a semistructured setting). What this may mean for you and your child is that you may want to plan to have ancillary assistance or more time available if your child is coming out of the hospital to supervise him or her at home. Many of my parents have worked out reasonable agreements with their workplace under the Family and Medical Leave Act (details are available from the U.S. Department of Labor at its website, *www.dol.gov/esa/whd/fmla*).

What are the reasons for hospitalizing a child?

Practitioners decide on hospitalization based on a number of variables. I am most concerned when children are potentially dangerous either to themselves (such as being suicidal) or to others (including the threat to harm a sibling, parent, or peer). Other reasons for hospitalizing children include a rapidly deteriorating condition, inadequate resources to manage them safely at home or in the community, severe behavioral medication reaction, unstable eating disorders, or the inability to complete further comprehensive assessment on an outpatient basis (e.g., when we need to assess "false seizures").

If I thought my child needed this type of care, what would I do?

The method of getting your child hospitalized varies among regions. In most cases, if you are concerned about your child's condition, contact the treating practitioner. If your child suddenly becomes out of control or dangerous to himself or to others, you may be in the position of having to take your child to the nearest emergency room or local mental health crisis center. If your child refuses to comply, you must seriously consider contacting the local police and ambulance to transport the child to the nearest evaluation site.

What happens when we get to the hospital?

In the crisis center or emergency room, your child will be assessed for hospitalization. If your child is deemed dangerous to herself or others, the practitioner may commit the child to a psychiatric hospital or psychiatric wing of the medical center. This commitment will last for an initial 3 days, during which the hospital, in collaboration with the child's caregivers, will determine the necessity of continuing hospital care. During the admitting process, you will be asked to voluntarily sign your child in to the psychiatric facility. You should stay with your child throughout the evaluation process and transfer to the psychiatric hospital. You can be very helpful in aiding your child in the transition to the hospital as well as providing invaluable information to the admitting team.

Does insurance cover psychiatric hospitalization of children?

Depending on your insurance, the decision to pay for hospitalization may need to be reviewed with the evaluation team prior to transfer to a hospital. Likewise, the specific hospital to which your child will be admitted may also be determined by your insurance and bed availability. If your insurance refuses to pay for the hospitalization, you may pay privately or your child may be sent to a state facility. If your child's hospitalization has been approved by the managed care reviewers, the hospital will need to provide evidence of the need for ongoing hospitalization. I suggest keeping in touch with both the hospital and your child's managed care company to know the status of your child's stay. If you or the hospital disagree with the length of stay approved, take advantage of the appeal process available to you.

How long will my child remain in the hospital?

It depends on the child's condition, the child and family's compliance with the process, outpatient resources, and the hospital. During my training in the early 1990s, juveniles were often hospitalized for 1–2 months. More recently, hospitalizations average 1–3 weeks. Your child may be transferred from intensive inpatient status to day treatment. Day treatment encompasses having your child spend nights and weekends at home while going to the hospital during the day. Many of the specifics of the approach to your child's care are based on the available resources, the outpatient provider's suggestions, and the amount and level of care provided by your child's insurance.

Will the hospital be able to figure out why my child's condition worsened?

Having your child in the hospital affords the opportunity, while in a safe environment, to get an initial or fresh comprehensive view of the situation. For instance, in certain cases I request an independent evaluation of my patient's diagnosis and current pharmacological approach. I often take advantage of a hospitalization by initiating a medication trial while the child is in this safe environment and can be monitored carefully for behavioral and medical complications.

How can I make this process productive for my child?

To facilitate your child's treatment, be sure that the hospital team is in contact with your child's outpatient team. Make yourselves available for individual and family meetings. Provide information on your child upon request. Also be sure to familiarize yourself with the hospital policy on bringing in toys or food, visitation, and phone calls.

How can I stop feeling so awful about this?

Be ready for a flood of emotions. Hospitalizing your child is one of the most conflictual experiences you will ever undergo. First and foremost, though, know that if your child is threatening suicide, you are doing the right thing to take that threat seriously and take action to protect your child. Some parents, probably out of fear of the reality of the situation, believe their children are only trying to get attention and may even try to talk their children out of feeling suicidal. This situation demands expert advice and may be urgent, in which case a hospital is a good source of help.

Added to the angst of the precipitating event leading to hospitalization, parents often experience guilt, separation anxiety, and helplessness (lack of control). Don't be surprised if you feel angry, sad, anxious, or detached while your child is hospitalized. Parents of my patients note that the support of friends and family is helpful during this time. Parents also report that seeing their own or their child's therapist or talking with the hospital social worker can be very educating, comforting, and supportive. They also report the additional stress of providing for their other children while worrying, visiting, and working with the various systems (such as insurance and school) that need to be in place for their hospitalized child to be discharged. Try to avoid tunneling your angst into the system unnecessarily. Although there are often many culprits who have not adequately assisted in the overall care of your child, try to use your energy constructively in setting up a new comprehensive strategy for your child. In summary, hospitalization is a trying process that can be used effectively in the care of your child.

PART II

Common Childhood Psychiatric Disorders

This section describes the most common emotional, behavioral, and developmental disorders seen in children and adolescents. Because every child is unique and so many have more than one disorder, your child is unlikely to fit snugly into any one of these molds. You may, however, find it helpful to consult these summaries of symptoms and behavior patterns during the diagnostic evaluation. Does the picture of the disorder in this book mesh with what you see in your child and what the practitioner is reporting to you? If not, what you read here may help you formulate questions that will push the evaluation process toward an accurate hypothesis.

You may also wish to come back to this section if you notice a change in your child's behavior or other symptoms. Could a new problem be developing? Are these signs typical of the child's disorder at the older age your child has reached? What is the disorder's expected course?

The fundamental information in the following chapters should serve as a springboard for the ongoing dialogue between you and the doctor that will ensure continued good care for your child. In addition to a description of symptoms and some examples of how

the various syndromes look in real children, each chapter tells
you what we know to date about neurological and other biological
causes. Following the description of each disorder, you will find
information on how we currently treat it—including methods for
resolving the side effects of some treatments—and why. Full descriptions of the pharmacological agents used in treatment are
given in Part III.

CHAPTER 5

ATTENTIONAL AND DISRUPTIVE BEHAVIORAL DISORDERS

ATTENTION-DEFICIT/HYPERACTIVITY DISORDER

Attention-deficit/hyperactivity disorder (ADHD) is the most common psychiatric disorder that pediatricians, family physicians, neurologists, and psychiatrists treat in children. It affects from 5 to 9% of school-age children, at least 70% of whom will continue to have the disorder into adolescence. About half of ADHD children will still have the disorder as adults. With age, the hyperactivity and impulsivity tend to diminish; however, the attentional problems persist.

The Disorder

In the past you may have heard basically the same syndrome called hyperkinesis disorder of childhood, minimal brain dysfunction, attention deficit disorder (ADD), ADDH, or ADD with or without hyperactivity. Today the disorder is known collectively as ADHD, as defined in the *DSM-IV-TR* (see page 70). The symptoms that characterize ADHD are inattentiveness, distractibility, impulsivity, and often hyperactivity, all to a degree considered inappropriate for the developmental stage of the child. That is, a 4-year-old who "can't sit still" would not necessarily be suspected of having ADHD. A 12-year-old with the same problem, however, would be suspect. Typically, ADHD children also have a low tolerance for frustration, shift activities frequently, get bored easily, are disorganized, and daydream a lot. Because ADHD reveals itself in atypical ways of feeling, thinking, and acting, it is known as an emotional, cognitive, and behavioral disorder.

The symptoms of ADHD are usually pervasive—they show up in many situations over a span of a few months—but they may not all occur in all settings. Children whose main problem is inattention, for example, may have difficulties in school and in completing homework but few troubles with peers or family. Children with more hyperactive or impulsive symptoms may do relatively well in school but have difficulties at home or in situations offering less guidance and structure. The symptoms of ADHD may impair the child's academic performance, overall behavior, and social/interpersonal relationships. But because the symptoms vary among children and in different environments, the disorder is not always easy to diagnose, especially when inattention is the predominant symptom.

Fifteen-year-old Steve, for instance, was doing worse and worse in school, taking an inordinate amount of time to complete homework, and becoming more and more frustrated and depressed. But cognitive (thinking ability) tests showed his intelligence was above-average, and he had no learning disabilities. It took a complete evaluation to reveal that Steve was highly inattentive and distractible, was unable to finish tasks, and was daydreaming a great deal of the time. After treatment with Ritalin sustained-release 20 mg in the morning, his inattention improved and so did his school performance. In turn, his self-esteem rose, and his frustration dropped over the next few months.

It can take some digging to unveil ADHD when the more noticeable symptoms of hyperactivity don't appear, but it is crucial that parents and other adults in the child's life not ignore symptoms like Steve's. Many children with untreated ADHD not only become dejected and discouraged by the problems their disorder imposes but begin to have other secondary problems as well.

Research shows that ADHD commonly occurs with oppositional defiant disorder (40–60% of cases) and conduct disorder (10–20%). More recent studies show that ADHD also occurs along with mood—depression and bipolar disorder (10–20%)—and anxiety disorders (35%). Learning disorders appear to co-occur with ADHD in up to one-third of children, so they should be suspected in all ADHD kids. If your child has specific learning problems in distinct academic areas such as reading, writing, or math, be sure to seek further evaluation—your child's school or pediatrician should be able to provide a referral.

The majority of basic science investigations indicate that ADHD is related to disturbances in the neurotransmitters dopamine and norepinephrine (but not in serotonin, another neurotransmitter you may have read a lot about). That is why you may hear ADHD called a neuropsychiatric disorder. These chemicals appear to be deficient in specific regions of the brain.

Very recently, researchers have turned their attention to certain other neurochemicals in the brain that may be related to ADHD, specifically acetylcholine and nicotine, two compounds that belong to the family of neurotransmitters called the *cholinergic system*. These neurotransmitters are concentrated in areas of the brain related to ADHD, including the attention and memory centers. Interestingly, much of the research with the cholinergic family comes from the following observations: ADHD children, adolescents, and adults are twice as likely to smoke cigarettes as their peers; maternal smoking during gestation may be a risk factor for ADHD in the unborn child; and cholinergic medications are effective in treating memory problems in adults (Alzheimer's disease). Research on drugs that work on the cholinergic system is under way in ADHD individuals. Some evidence suggests that medications used to improve thinking processes in Alzheimer's patients (e.g., Reminyl) may also improve specific thinking processes in ADHD, such as organization.

Brain imaging used in research has shown that certain parts of the brain are usually different in ADHD individuals: the frontal lobes; the striatum, which is rich in dopamine; the cingulate, involved in attention, emotions, and memory; and the corpus collosum, which is the major connection among the lobes of the brain. Brain scanning has in fact confirmed what neuropsychology has discovered: that these are the areas related to attention, vigilance, and distractibility. Research over the years since this book was first published is beginning to reveal a lot about the genetic basis of ADHD. For instance, children with ADHD have been found to have a few different types of problems with their genes that are linked to subtle, but important, problems in nerve-to-nerve communication.

Despite the neurological causes of ADHD, brain activity and brain imaging tests such as EEGs; brain electrical activity mapping, or BEAMs (fancy EEGs); and single-photon-emission space tomography, or SPECT (blood flow) studies are *not* considered reliable or valid in diagnosing ADHD; nor are blood tests. To date, a comprehensive history of the problem remains the best way to identify the disorder. The neuropsychological tests used in research studies—the CPT (Continuous Performance Test),

Wisconsin Card Sort, Stroop Test, and TOVA—are also *not* part of the standard clinical evaluation for ADHD. There simply are not enough scientific data to support their effectiveness in diagnosing ADHD or directing medication management in day-to-day clinical practice. If an evaluator suggests such tests, therefore, you would be wise to ask why and consider another practitioner.

If your child was diagnosed with ADHD since the publication of the most recent revision of the *DSM* (*DSM-IV-TR* [2000]), he or she should have been diagnosed as having either the hyperactive subtype, the inattentive subtype, or the combined subtype. But diagnostic classification and criteria for ADHD seem to be in an ongoing state of flux as we learn more about the course of this disorder and its different manifestations. As of this revision, approximately one-half of pediatric referrals (one-quarter of psychiatric) have the inattentive subtype of ADHD. But controversy exists over whether it is really intimately related to the combined subtype. For example, inattentives have less co-occurring difficulties, perhaps a different cognitive style (sluggish), and less overall impairment. Do kids who shed the predominate hyperactivity/impulsivity as they grow up really have the inattentive subtype, or are they really grown-ups with combined subtype ADHD? In general, the medication response for stimulants and nonstimulants is similar between the subtypes. In other words, kids with the inattentive subtype respond as well to the stimulants and nonstimulants as those who have the more classic "combined" subtype.

Also, it used to be thought that girls were overrepresented in the inattentive subtype, but that no longer appears to be true. Recent information on girls with ADHD indicate that they often internalize much of the stigma yet share many of the same characteristics and co-occurring problems that boys with the disorder have. For example, medications work equally well in girls and boys with ADHD.

The Treatment

Medication is considered one of the most important treatments for ADHD. In fact, its use with this disorder has been studied more extensively than any other application of psychopharmacology in children. One recent large study in children with ADHD and without other disorders completed in New York and Montreal demonstrated that, compared to intensive multimodal treatment including medications and psychotherapy, properly prescribed stimulants alone had the greatest positive effect after 2 years. Another very important study, funded by the National Institute of

Mental Health, produced similar results, showing that medications were superior to behavioral treatments alone for the core symptoms of ADHD. The study also found that behavioral treatment along with medication management was the most effective treatment to address some of the noncore symptoms (self-esteem, peer relationships, family functioning, and social skills).

> **multimodal treatment**: The use of two or more different distinct types of therapy (such as medications and psychotherapy).

Stimulant medications—notably Ritalin (methylphenidate), Ritalin LA (extended-release methylphenidate), Metadate CD Focalin, Concerta (extended-release methylphenidate), Adderall (amph   Adderall XR (extended-release amphetamine), and Dexedrine   amine)—are the best-studied class of drugs for ADHD, a   they are the treatment of choice. Stimulants generally w   immediately when the correct dose is achieved. Although it is unusual for children to develop a tolerance to these drugs, children may need increasing doses as they grow.

Practitioners have found that if one stimulant is unsuccessful it is worth trying another, but if your child cannot tolerate the stimulants or has prominent anxiety or tics, Strattera (atomoxetine) should be tried. Strattera is a recently FDA approved nonstimulant noradrenergic medication that is very useful for ADHD. Strattera usually takes a few weeks to see its full benefit and is sometimes used with stimulants.

Second-line treatments include the antidepressants, both the tricyclics (desipramine, imipramine, nortriptyline) and Wellbutrin. Although you may see an effect immediately, antidepressants may take up to 4 weeks to reach full effectiveness. As with the stimulants, if one antidepressant is not effective, your child's doctor would be wise to try another.

For children as young as 3–5, or in aggressive or especially overactive kids, the blood pressure medications (antihypertensives) Catapres (clonidine) and Tenex (guanfacine) may be useful. These drugs may also help with the sleep problems that sometimes plague children with ADHD or that result from its treatment, such as using Concerta or Adderall.

Some medications that are still being tested for ADHD are Provigil (modafinil) and a class of medications called the *cholinesterase inhibitors* (Aricept [donpezil], Reminyl [galantamine], Exelon [rivastigmine]). Provigil is not a stimulant medication but is a medication that is FDA approved for narcolepsy. Termed a wake-promoting agent, Provigil has had mixed results in large trials for ADHD in adults. At a dose of approximately 200 mg in the morning and 100 mg in the afternoon, a large multisite study indicated a moderate response in reducing ADHD symptoms with minimal side effects (most commonly headaches, stomachaches, edginess, insomnia). My experience is that for kids with ADHD who do not respond to traditional agents Provigil may be helpful.

The cholinesterase medications are approved for use in Alzheimer's disorder to slow down the deterioration in memory dysfunction. These medications have been of interest in that they may assist in nonspecific cognitive operations as well as more specifically assisting in executive operations of the brain such as planning, organization, project execution, followthrough, and so on. Our experience and preliminary data indicate that these agents may take up to 3 months to see an effect and may be associated with nausea, diarrhea, and dizziness.

Do not be surprised if your child's doctor ends up prescribing a combination of medications, such as Ritalin with desipramine, Wellbutrin and stimulants, or stimulants with clonidine. That is the way we often get the best possible improvement in ADHD symptoms. More than one drug may also be necessary if your child, like about half of the children who have ADHD, has other psychiatric disorders as well. Naturally comorbidity (see page 20) complicates treatment. Atomoxetine may be particularly useful as monotherapy (single medication) in comorbid ADHD with tics, anxiety, or depression.

- In children with ADHD and anxiety disorders, the stimulants may worsen the anxiety, in which case atomoxetine or a tricyclic antidepressant such as nortriptyline, another antidepressant (including Wellbutrin, Effexor, or Serzone), or an antihypertensive may be helpful. Your child's doctor may need to combine agents such as a medication for ADHD plus one for anxiety such as Buspar or a Valium-like agent.
- For children with ADHD and depression, the use of atomoxetine or an antidepressant such as Wellbutrin, a tricyclic antidepressant (imipramine, desipramine, etc.), or Effexor may be effective on its own. Or, as documented by the experience of many clinicians and one research report, the Prozac-like medications (SSRIs) along with the stimulants could work. Fifteen-year-old Sara, already tak-

ing Metadate CD (methylphenidate extended release) for ADHD, did very well with 20 mg of Paxil daily and 20 mg daily of Metadate CD after the depression she had developed failed to respond to changing medications and psychotherapy.

- Children with bipolar disorder and ADHD can be treated with an antipsychotic or a mood stabilizer for the bipolar disorder and a stimulant, antihypertensive, or a tricyclic antidepressant for the ADHD. Recent data in adults suggest Wellbutrin is a good choice for severe moodiness plus ADHD.

- The sizable group of children and adolescents with mental retardation or developmental disorders with prominent ADHD symptoms may also benefit from pharmacological treatment of the ADHD. Although untested scientifically, there has been some interest in the use of Strattera for kids with ADHD and Asperger syndrome or pervasive developmental disorder. Clinicians have reported improved ADHD symptoms, improved socialization and interaction, and less anxiety.

- It is important to realize, however, that the care of specific developmental disorders including learning disabilities is largely remedial and supportive. That is, medications don't treat the mental retardation or learning disabilities but may help remedial treatment to work better.

- Children with ADHD who have prominent organizational and time-management issues (executive function problems) may benefit from a medicine for their ADHD plus an Alzheimer's medication (e.g., Aricept, Exelon, Reminyl).

Whatever medications end up being prescribed, when you should give them to your child depends on the severity and pervasiveness of the child's problems and relies largely on your judgment. Most children should remain on their medication all the time. However, your child may need the drug only during school, with weekend and vacation holidays off the medication, or around the clock and on vacations. If, for example, your child has made lasting friendships only since being placed on a stimulant, you probably won't want to limit the medication to school hours. But for a child whose main problem is inattention at school, weekend and vacation holidays may be fine. Whereas the stimulants can be discontinued on weekends, it is advisable not to change the dosing of Strattera (atomoxetine) or the antidepressants.

OPPOSITIONAL DEFIANT DISORDER

Eleven-year-old Tim snaps at his mother when limits are set, argues incessantly, and frequently uses foul language. He instigates trouble among his siblings but is quick to blame them for problems for which he is clearly responsible. Tim is typical of children with oppositional defiant disorder. He creates problems for his family and others, although he doesn't inflict major harm, damage property, or steal.

The Disorder

Like Tim, children with oppositional defiant disorder are extremely difficult to care for or be around because their ongoing behavior falls at the extreme end of normal on a continuum. Parents and other adults often bear the brunt of the child's behavior since the child's oppositionality is usually directed at authority figures. They often appear inflexible and have a quick temper in response to limit setting. While children who have oppositional defiant disorder will not necessarily be depressed, they will appear to have a pretty consistently negative attitude, taking the opposite side against you, teachers, or other authority figures, being quick to blame others for their behavior, frequently swearing, acting like "tough guys," and being annoying to or being annoyed easily by others. The good news is that a large group of these children grow out of the disorder as they become young adults. The bad news is that a small group will progress to conduct disorder, generally by a young age (see page 151).

No specific brain region has been implicated in oppositional defiant disorder, although disruption in serotonin may be involved in those who are oppositional and aggressive.

The Treatment

If your child also has ADHD or a mood disorder, as is common with oppositional defiant disorder, the medications for the former may reduce the intensity of the oppositionality as well. The antihypertensives clonidine and Tenex, the stimulants, Strattera, the tricyclics, or Wellbutrin also may reduce some of the symptoms and impairment associated with the disorder, but to date no one has found one single agent that effectively treats primary oppositional defiant disorder (oppositionality that does not stem from another disorder). Risperdal (and presumably the other atypical antipsychotics) has been shown to be effective in more severe cases typically associated with conduct disorder (see below). Fortunately, medication is not your only option—behavioral modification appears to help both parents and children develop strategies for managing and reducing the impact of the symptoms.

CONDUCT DISORDER

The Disorder

What mental health professionals of today call *conduct disorder* has often been viewed informally as juvenile delinquency—behavior that consistently violates the basic rights of others and disregards societal norms and rules. Bullying of younger children, cruelty to animals, fights, sometimes with weapons, and purposeful destruction of property are common among children with conduct disorder. The stealing, truancy, and lying that occasionally appear in normal development are rampant and persistent in the child with conduct disorder. A hallmark of conduct disorder is lack of remorse for these problematic behaviors or refusal to take responsibility for them.

Children with conduct disorder are usually very aggressive. Some have uncontrolled outbursts and may be described as having a bad temper; their outbursts may be triggered by individual external events or related to having some psychiatric disturbance such as a mood problem like bipolar disorder. Others behave in a more predatory fashion, and their behavior may come across as cold, callous, and premeditated.

The Treatment

In some cases, conduct disorder appears to be passed on from parent to child, especially to the sons of alcoholic and antisocial fathers. Despite the fact that serotonin levels have been found to be lower and EEG activity may be different in conduct-disordered children and aggressive adults, pharmacotherapy has not proved to be a very satisfactory treatment. Children with the outburst type of aggression may respond more favorably to pharmacological intervention than those who perform calculated aggressive acts. But medication seems most likely to help when it is used to treat a co-occurring problem, such as depression or bipolar disorder. One study found that children with conduct disorder and depression who took imipramine had a substantial reduction in both their conduct symptoms and their depression. Similar findings were reported in ADHD youth with conduct disorder who were treated with methylphenidate. Aggressiveness shared by youth with conduct and bipolar disorder is reduced significantly with the atypical antipsychotics (e.g., Risperdal, Zyprexa). As of the revision of this book, Risperdal (risperidone) was about to receive FDA approval for children and adolescents with "disruptive disorders" (oppositional and conduct disorder).

If you suspect that your child has conduct disorder, then be sure to ask your doctor to look for other conditions: not only depression and bipolar disorder but also ADHD, posttraumatic stress, or anxiety. These disorders respond not only to pharmacological intervention but also to psychotherapy.

In the final analysis, intermittent treatment with behavioral and family therapy may be necessary for both the child and the family. Studies indicate that most children will continue to have the disorder, or aggressivity, for a long time. Long-term information indicates that an intact family may be one of the most important factors in the eventual positive outcome of the grown-up child with conduct disorder.

TABLE 5. Pharmacotherapy of ADHD and the Disruptive Behavioral Disorders

Disorder	Pharmacotherapy
Attention-deficit/ hyperactivity disorder (ADHD)	Stimulants—Ritalin, Dexedrine, Adderall, Concerta First-line drugs of choice (FDA-approved) Extended-release preparations preferred (Concerta, Ritalin LA, Metadate CD) Caution in patients with tics or marked height/weight problems Strattera (atomoxetine) First-line agent (FDA-approved) May be particularly useful in comorbid cases Caution with bipolar disorder Cylert Caution with liver problems Clonidine, Tenex (guanfacine) Good for overactivity and impulsivity, preschoolers First line for patients with ADHD + tics Tricyclic antidepressants—desipramine, nortriptyline, imipramine Second line after stimulants/Strattera Good for co-occurring depression, anxiety, or tics Caution if cardiac problems Wellbutrin (bupropion) Second line after stimulants/Strattera Caution if tics or seizures May be useful for comorbid depression or bipolar disorder Combined pharmacotherapy for resistant cases
Conduct disorder, oppositional defiant disorder (ODD)	No specific pharmacotherapy available for core disorders Look for and treat other disorders (e.g., bipolar disorder, depression) Consider stimulants, Strattera, antidepressants (tricyclics or Wellbutrin) For agitation, aggression, and self-abuse Beta blockers (e.g., propranolol) Clonidine, guanfacine Benzodiazepines (e.g., Valium, Klonopin) Lithium, anticonvulsants (e.g., Tegretol, Valproate, Trileptal, Neurontin) Naltrexone Antipsychotics (e.g., Seroquel, Risperdal, Thorazine, Mellaril, Zyprexa)

CHAPTER 6

AUTISM AND PERVASIVE DEVELOPMENTAL DISORDERS

Children vary widely in their mental and physical development over time. A small group have what we call *developmental disorders*—either substantial delays in reaching developmental milestones or failure to reach those milestones. A child can have a developmental disorder in a very specific area such as a problem with reading (developmental reading disorder), writing (developmental writing disorder), or processing verbal information (central auditory information processing disorder). Or the developmental disorder can be more global, affecting learning (mental retardation), emotions, or speech and language (autism and pervasive developmental disorder). Whereas a child who is speaking few words by age 2 may be within normal development, a similar problem in a 7-year-old flags a major problem.

THE DISORDERS

Autism and the pervasive developmental disorders (PDDs) are characterized by marked impairment in several areas of development, but what parents might find most noticeable and most disturbing is the child's apparent disconnection from the rest of the world. Many parents describe children with PDDs as "living in their head" or "inhabiting their own little world." These children may seem distant, unemotional, passive, and withdrawn. Many parents report that their children seemed unresponsive to emotional interactions, cold, and aloof as early as infancy or toddlerhood. Mental health professionals now believe that these disorders do begin in early childhood; autism probably is present prenatally and seems to have a prominent genetic component.

> **occupational therapy**: A type of therapy that helps children regain the basic tools necessary to function. Kids work on using their hands to improve dexterity, doing coordination exercises and expressing themselves with art.

Autistic children and children with PDDs often have very restricted interactive social skills. They simply don't seem to reciprocate or connect with others. Delayed or essentially nonexistent speech and language communication are very common, as is poor nonverbal communication. Children with PDDs often don't make eye contact and can't read or interpret social cues, from smiles or expressions of anger to the more complicated "body language."

These children generally have a limited repertoire of interests and activities, and some have a very active fantasy life. Though no one knows why, changes in their routine and surprises often elicit anger and anxiety in children and adolescents with pervasive developmental disorders.

Children with pervasive developmental disorder often engage in repetitive actions, commonly called *stereotypic behaviors,* that seem bizarre to onlookers. This behavior may include rocking, hair twirling, biting themselves, and head banging. Sometimes the stereotypic behavior is set off by the anxiety of a change in routine; often the child is apparently trying to stimulate herself. Again, we don't know exactly what is at work in stereotypic behavior.

Some children, like 13-year-old Ralph, have a more unusual developmental disorder often called *Asperger syndrome.* Ralph has long-standing ADHD but normal speech and language development. He does relatively well academically but has no friends or interest in making any. Ralph is very interested in police vehicles and spends his free time hanging out with the police and listening to their calls. Ralph's condition is known as a "high functioning pervasive developmental disorder" because his disturbances are mainly in social interactions and are more isolated than in autism or PDD, allowing him to function more easily in his world. Metadate CD improved Ralph's ADHD symptoms, and occupational therapy during elementary school has helped him function better. As he has matured, his ability to get along with his peers has improved too. However, the difficulty in having and maintaining friendships can hit hard in adolescence, bringing on demoralization and depression. So, if your child is diagnosed with Asperger syndrome, talk to the doctor about how to watch for depression.

In the past, disorders like autism were thought to be caused in part by cold, aloof parenting. Now scientists agree that no specific parenting or environmental factor appears to cause PDDs. Scientific reports based on brain imaging pictures have suggested instead that abnormal neurological development is at the root of the problem. Multiple regions of the brain, including the size of the fluid cavities of the brain (ventricles), appear to be different in children with developmental disorders. Lower serotonin levels have also been reported in these children. Because children with these disorders may also have excessive anxiety and obsessiveness, depression, bipolar disorder, psychosis, and ADHD, it is important that the doctor carefully evaluate your child for co-occurring disorders. The child's daily functioning stands a good chance of improving once other problems are identified and treated.

Autism, Asperger sydrome, and PDDs affect only about 30 of every 10,000 children, but still this is a 50% increase in incidence over the past few decades. This increase has raised considerable controversy: Why has there been such a huge increase in diagnosis of these developmental disorders? Are we overdiagnosing these disorders? Also being debated are the appropriate interventions and the claims about cause on which they are based: the use of diet and other peripheral treatments. Of note, there is a much higher incidence of gastrointestinal problems in individuals affected with autism, and this is currently an area of intensive scientific study. A large multisite study recently demonstrated that risperidone was highly effective in reducing autistic symptoms and self-injury. Recent work with cholinesterase inhibitors (Reminyl, Aricept, Exelon) suggest that these agents may be selectively very helpful in assisting these children with general cognition. In contrast, gastrin, secretin, and other peptide hormones that were supposed to be helpful in controlled trials failed.

The Treatment

Behavior therapy continues to be the most popular nonpharmacological strategy for pervasive developmental disorder and autism. There is no specific standard medication regimen, so prepare yourself to be patient through the trial-and-error process that treatment of PDD often demands. However, medications can be very helpful in diminishing some of the core symptoms of the PDD/autism, such as rigidity and anxiety. Twelve-year-old Chaka is a fairly typical example. Brought to me for help with the self-biting that accompanied her autism, she also would self-stimulate herself by rocking and occasionally required a helmet as well because of her head banging against the wall when her routine was changed. Her eye contact was limited, her speech development poor, and she engaged in little non-verbal communication. Physically she appeared immature, had small underdeveloped ears, and her eyes were close together. We tried Trexane, Depakote, Inderal, clonidine, and Klonopin, all to no avail, despite their reported effectiveness in many cases. Finally she responded moderately well to Zoloft, the antidepressant that belongs to the selective serotonin reuptake inhibitors (SSRIs) increasingly used for these children.

While sometimes remarkably helpful, the problem with Zoloft and other individual drugs is that they reduce only some of the core symptoms and therefore cannot entirely resolve the impairment caused by autism or PDD. The SSRIs Zoloft, Prozac, Paxil, Lexapro, Celexa, and Luvox, in addition to a tricyclic antidepressant called Anafranil, reduce the obsessive and compulsive activity, rigidity, anxiety, and irritability that often accompany pervasive developmental disorder and autism. They are not especially useful, however, with the communication or social interaction problems. Strattera has been reported by some clinicians to be helpful in reducing the anxiety and improving the socialization in some kids with autism spectrum disorders.

Two classes of medications, the antihypertensives and the atypical antipsychotics, also can be helpful for certain behaviors associated with the developmental disorders. Although they didn't work for Chaka, beta blockers such as propranolol at generally high doses (up to 240 mg per day) and clonidine (typically dosed 0.1 mg three to four times daily) are increasingly reported to be useful in controlling the aggression of developmentally disordered patients, whether that aggression is directed at themselves (head banging or self-mutilating behavior) or others. Older work with Haldol and more recent work with Risperdal (risperidone) has demonstrated their usefulness for youth with PDD. In a large multisite study of Risperdal, not only did the symptoms of PDD improve, but there was a notable improvement in functioning. I treat Justin, a 7-year-old with ADHD, some mood concerns, and PDD. He had outbursts limiting his participation in mainstream classes that were unresponsive to ADHD treatment and SSRIs. Low-dose Risperdal (0.5 mg) was extremely helpful in controlling his outbursts (usually secondary to frustration), and he is doing well in a regular classroom with additional support.

Self-mutilating behavior can sometimes be reduced by using nal-trexone or Rivea at doses of 25 mg up to three times daily.

Children with pervasive developmental disorders have a lot of problems with cognition and executive function. As described on page 34, executive functioning is like the secretary of the brain (or the function of the mother or father!)—helping the child organize, plan, execute, and follow through on a project. Obviously, executive function deficits make it extremely difficult for a child to conduct a normal life. Recent research has produced some preliminary data suggesting that cholinesterase inhibitors (Reminyl, Aricept, Exelon) may be selectively very helpful in assisting these children with general cognition and executive function in particular, but since little research is currently being conducted, it could be a long time before such medications become accepted for this use. In contrast, gastrin and secretin and other peptides that were supposed to be helpful to children with PDD failed when tested in controlled trials.

For children who have severe irritability, moodiness, or depression, the antidepressants already mentioned may be helpful. And if the child's mood swings are substantial, a mood-stabilizing agent such as lithium, Tegretol, Trileptal, Depakote, Neurontin, or Lamictal may be beneficial. In children with prominent anxiety symptoms such as around mealtimes, the Valium-like medications (benzodiazepines) such as Ativan and Klonopin may be useful. Children with PPD/autism and ADHD or prominent ADHD-like symptoms benefit from the same medications for ADHD, namely stimulants, antidepressants, and antihypertensives. It is notable that many children with PPD or autism also have a seizure disorder and require an anticonvulsant. If your child is one of them, you need to talk to the doctor about potential drug interactions with other medications used to address behavioral concerns.

In November 2003, the U.S. federal government unveiled a 10-year interagency plan to address the growing rate of autistic disorders in American children. Goals target coordinated biomedical research, earlier diagnosis, and therapeutic methods. A goal listed as realistic in the plan is to develop effective treatments along with the Department of Education. One that is currently considered more challenging is the development of effective drugs for these disorders. Because this is a long-term plan that is still very unformed, it will probably be years before results begin to appear, but parents should watch for news of these promising efforts.

TABLE 6. Pharmacotherapy of Autism and Pervasive
Developmental Disorders

No specific pharmacotherapy for the core disorder

Look for other disorders (ADHD, depression, anxiety)

Pharmacotherapy of repetitive behaviors
    Selective and nonselective serotonin reuptake inhibitors—Prozac, Zoloft,
      Luvox, Paxil, Anafranil, Celexa, Lexapro
    Atypical antipsychotics (e.g., Risperdal, Zyprexa, Seroquel, Geodon, Abilify)

For aggression and self-abuse
    Beta blockers (e.g., propranolol) Clonidine, Tenex
    Benzodiazepines (e.g., Klonopin, Tranxene)
    Lithium, anticonvulsants (i.e., Tegretol, Valproate, Neurontin, Trileptal),
      Naltrexone

CHAPTER 7

THE MOOD DISORDERS

Many parents who bring children to our clinic because of "emotional problems" end up describing what mental health professionals term *mood disorders*. Mood is generally considered your child's ongoing emotional state, and any disturbance in that state that lasts continually for more than 2 weeks or occurs for most of the day over a substantial period of time should be evaluated as a possible mood disorder.

Mood disorders in children are classified in two principal ways: (1) as depression alone or bipolar disorder (also called manic–depression) and (2) as major or minor. You are probably familiar with the most typical symptoms of depression: sadness, gloominess, loss of interest and enjoyment in life. When a child's "moodiness" falls generally into those categories, the child is likely to be diagnosed with depression. But when emotional symptoms that seem the opposite of depression also appear— euphoria or severe irritability, explosive energy, racing thoughts, and extremely goal-directed actions—bipolar disorder is usually suspected. (Complicating diagnosis, however, is that depression often manifests itself in children as irritability or anger instead of sadness.) These "high" or "severely agitated" symptoms are called *mania,* and their contrast with "lows" or depression results in the term *bipolar* (meaning two poles of mood).

A mood disorder is considered major or minor based on its severity and course over time. Major mood disorders affecting children include major depression and bipolar disorder. Other mood disorders include a less severe form of depression called *dysthymia.* Commonly mistaken for a personality or character flaw, dysthymia should be taken quite seriously because it can be very damaging to a child's quality of life. Dysthymia is very long-standing—often more than 2 years in duration. It does not involve full-blown depression, but the child may have a long-term negative and irritable mood, appearing constantly unhappy, low in energy, and uninterested in activity. Not surprisingly, the child may have problems with friends and classmates and with parents and siblings. All of this can damage the child's self-esteem over the 2 years or more that dysthymia is likely to last. Often the disorder is a precursor of more severe depression that begins later in adolescence or adulthood.

One reason that depressive disorders can be so injurious to children is that both depression and manic depression tend to be long-standing (chronic) with only infrequent spontaneous remissions, compared to the adult forms, which tend to cycle. Another is that these disorders in children can be difficult to diagnose, especially depression. It is not always easy to see that a child has been "down" for an extended period of time. Maybe your son isn't very forthcoming about how he's feeling; perhaps your daughter is too young to articulate her moods clearly. Consider, too, that children often seem moody, sometimes due to passing external pressures (e.g., losing a sport event, peer difficulties) and sometimes due to transitions in their maturation. We've all known preteens and teens who seem pretty constantly crabby or glum, and it's difficult to determine when they're just "going through a phase" and when they're suffering from clinical depression and need help. Finally, we tend to view "real" depression as an adult disease and don't often make the connection between less obvious symptoms—fatigue and listlessness, irritability, lack of concentration—and a mood disorder. Fourteen-year-old Donny, for example, was referred to us by his pediatrician because the doctor could find no medical illness to account for his low energy level. It took a psychiatric evaluation to find out that Donny could not report the last time he had been happy, that he felt blue and cynical "all the time," and to observe that he was quiet and withdrawn. When we do evaluate children for mood disorders, we often find—as we did in Donny's case—that the child's problems began as long as a year or two ago.

As a parent, you can be guided to some extent by the fact that the rate of depression increases with age. Major depression is estimated to affect 0.3% of preschoolers, 1–2% of elementary-age children, and 5% of adolescents. In other words, the younger your child is, the less likely she is to be suffering from major depression. Until adolescence, roughly the same number of boys and girls suffer from depression. Then the more typical adult pattern starts with approximately two-thirds of cases affecting women. Depressive disorders commonly co-occur with anxiety, ADHD, conduct, and substance use disorders in older children and adolescents.

DEPRESSION

The Disorder

As already mentioned, depression in a child may appear as a sad or irritable mood or a continued loss of interest or pleasure in favorite activities. If you *ask* your child how *she* feels, however, it is important to know that children have difficulty distinguishing sad from mad or may report feeling sad and mad at the same time. Your observations may be more informative than the child's reporting to the practitioner. Be alert for school difficulties, refusal to attend school, withdrawal, isolation, physical complaints, negative attitude, frequent crying spells, and/or aggressive, antisocial behavior—all indications of possible depression in a child. The physical symptoms that many depressed adults have may also occur in a child: fatigue; changes in appetite and weight; abnormal sleep patterns (either too much or poor quality); physical slowing or agitation; and diminished ability to think. Depressed kids and teens may report feeling worthless, hopeless, trapped, guilty, or preoccupied with suicidal thoughts. Many are unable to think positively of the future. Severe depression may even include disturbances in reality (psychosis), most typically hearing voices (*auditory hallucinations*).

You can see why depression may be hard for parents to identify with any certainty. Both overconcern and underconcern can lead you astray. Unless you look carefully at the context of your child's moods, you may have trouble differentiating depression from temperament (such as a tendency toward temper tantrums) or passing emotions such as unhappiness or disappointment that commonly occur during childhood. A good distinguishing rule of thumb is that if the mood continues after the stressor that caused frustration or sadness has ended, the child *may* have a depressive disorder. Even if the symptoms do eventually end, a prolonged and exaggerated response, including many symptoms of depression, to a common stressor such as doing poorly on a test may indicate that the child is clinically depressed. As we discussed on pages 10–13 and 19–20, some children inherit the tendency toward depression, which is triggered by a certain stressor.

A child who has a full repertoire of depressive symptoms for at least 2 weeks is said to have a major depression. These symptoms may include irritability mixed with sadness, low energy and interest, somatic problems (stomachaches, headaches), crying spells, withdrawal, a sad expression, problems with concentrating, and thoughts about harming himself. Adolescents with major depression have more adult-like features to their depression and may have the following symptoms: irritability, cynicism, sadness, low energy and interest, crying spells, social isolation and withdrawal, concentration difficulties, and suicidality. No blood tests are used to diagnose any of the mood disorders in clinical practice. Psychological tests may be helpful in elucidating discrepancies in thinking and depressive themes in the interpretive parts of the test, but essentially mood disorders are diagnosed on the basis of the child's history of problems—symptoms, timing, and functioning.

As to the causes of depression, clearly there is a component that is passed on through families and thought to be genetic. From 30 to 50% of children with depression have a family member with depression. Likewise, the environment and excessive life stressors can cause a child to become depressed. As with many other disturbances in children and teenagers, the child probably has a genetic vulnerability to develop depression that becomes activated with stressors—a typical scenario in which genes and the environment interact. Medical causes may also underlie depression. Injuries to certain areas of the brain and some types of seizures may mimic or cause depression. Disturbances in thyroid hormone (both high and low) and drugs of abuse (such as cocaine and marijuana) can also cause depression in young people.

The Treatment

In general, juvenile-onset depression does not respond as well to treatment as adult depression. Psychotherapy continues to be the first line of treatment for mild to moderate depression, with medications used for moderate to severe depression. Probably all kids with moderate or severe depression should receive both medication and psychotherapy. Although traditional interpersonal and insight-oriented therapies can be helpful, more recently proactive, cognitive-based approaches that work on changing the child's perceptions and belief systems are gaining favor and have recently been proven effective. Be patient; these psychotherapies may take 2–3 months to start working. If your child refuses or is unable to engage in psychotherapy, medications should be considered. Likewise, if your child continues to have prominent mood problems despite a reasonable course (about 8–12 weeks) of psychotherapy, you should consider a medication consultation. Medication should be considered immediately in kids with previous depression (recurrent), suicidality, or severe depressive features with a lot of impairment.

The pharmacotherapy of depression in children and adolescents relies on the antidepressants. The most effective and commonly used agents in juvenile depression are the selective serotonin reuptake inhibitors (SSRIs), which include Zoloft, Prozac, Luvox, Lexapro, and Celexa. Studies of Prozac, Zoloft, and Celexa suggest their effectiveness in depression in kids.

These medications also appear particularly effective compared to the other antidepressants for the treatment of long-standing minor depression (dysthymia)—20 mg of Prozac was the prescription that helped 14-year-old Donny, introduced earlier. Note, however, that the study my group recently conducted with the makers of Prozac showed that 10 mg/day was sufficient for younger children. While we don't have similar studies of the other SSRIs, it seems prudent to start younger children on one-half of an adult starting dose.

Dosing of this class of medication is similar to that used in adults: Prozac or Celexa from 5 to 40 mg daily; Zoloft from 50 to 200 mg; Luvox from 50 to 300 mg. It is not uncommon to see an improvement in a child's state in the first week; however, it may take up to 12 weeks to know if the medication is going to work. Two years of psychotherapy had helped identify the triggers of 12-year-old Jeff's more severe depression, but the low energy and low interest, the sadness and sense of isolation that went along with his dysthymia persisted. Prozac resulted in Jeff's having a panic attack, so we tried Zoloft. At 75 mg daily, the Zoloft proved instrumental in reducing Jeff's depressive symptoms.

Other antidepressants commonly used for depression in children include Wellbutrin, Serzone, Remeron, trazodone, and the tricyclic antidepressants (desipramine, imipramine, amitriptyline, and others). At the time of printing, the efficacy of two new agents, atomoxetine and duloxetine, remains unclear in children with depression. Less commonly, the mood stabilizers (see below) are used for depression that features prominent mood swings, or lability.

---

lability: Rapid mood swings or moodiness.

When children exhibit depression and another disorder, the choice of a broader-spectrum agent that treats both disorders may be preferable. For children who have prominent ADHD and depression, Wellbutrin, the tricyclic antidepressants, or perhaps atomoxetine may be the initial drugs of choice. Children with anxiety and depression may be tried on an SSRI (a Prozac-like medication), a tricyclic antidepressant, Serzone, or trazodone. When none of the antidepressants seems to work, the doctor may try a higher dose of an antidepressant as long as the child is having no adverse effects from the antidepressants. Or a different class of medication may be prescribed. A third approach might be to combine two antidepressants of different classes (e.g., Celexa and desipramine), or an antidepressant with another medication, such as lithium, buspirone, stimulants, thyroid hormone, and anxiety-breaking medications.

Finding the right drug for your child leaves you and the doctor with the question of how long to treat the child, and unfortunately there is currently little information available to answer it. Often doctors are left relying on guidelines meant to apply to depressed adults. Because most adults' mood will improve naturally in 6 months to 1 year, for example, doctors tend to prescribe medication for 6–12 months. In children, however, depression frequently lasts longer and is less likely to remit spontaneously. The solution in our clinic is to continue medication for 1 year or longer, until the child's mood is stable for at least 3 months, and then very gradually taper the medication. If any symptoms of depression re-emerge, we know we need to consider restarting the medication or to boost the dosage to its original level. Often, though, we find we can reduce the maintenance dose of the medication.

We feel strongly that parents and children should *not* feel any pressure to stop the medication if they are concerned about a recurrence of the depression and will continue prescribing it upon request. In the earlier case of Jeff, who had been on Zoloft for 8 months, his parents and I agreed to continue the medication for another 4 months before reviewing discontinuance. In that case, the theoretical risks of long-term treatment were far outweighed by the real risk of depression and associated problems. This seems particularly pertinent in light of research showing that about half of adolescents with depression still have problems with their mood as adults and that long-term treatment of depression continues to lead to improved outcomes.

BIPOLAR (MANIC–DEPRESSIVE) DISORDER

The Disorder

Imagine feeling very depressed but at the same time very agitated and out of control. That, in a nutshell, is the "miserable feeling" that most children with bipolar or manic–depressive disorder and their parents describe. It reflects the intertwining of symptoms that distinguishes childhood manic depression from its adult counterpart. Where adults are likely to have broad mood swings, children with this problem typically experience both manic and depressive features at the same time, and the symptoms stay with the child for long periods.

In children, mania commonly takes the form of an extremely irritable or explosive mood, sometimes psychosis, with poor social interactions or functioning that is often devastating to the child and family. On top of the severe mood swings that make everyone's life difficult, the manic child may overflow with excess energy that makes it hard to sleep, propels the boy or girl into obsessively goal-directed activity, subjects the child to unrelenting racing thoughts, and turns the child into an overtalkative, loud dervish. Many of these children exhibit markedly poor judgment, pursuing thrill-seeking, reckless, or sex-based activities. Up to half of bipolar children have a relative with bipolar illness. Although mania in children should be differentiated from ADHD, conduct disorder, depression, and disturbances in reality (psychosis), these disorders commonly occur along with juvenile bipolar disorder. In fact, the younger the child with bipolar disorder, the more likely she is to have other psychiatric disorders.

As this revised edition goes to press, controversy simmers over juvenile bipolar disorder. Does the disorder really occur in children? Is it overdiagnosed? The incidence in children was unknown 5 years ago but today is reported to be anywhere from 1 to 5% of children. Also, is bipolar disorder a disorder with many related symptoms, or is it really the presence of co-occurring disorders (such as anxiety/panic disorder, ADHD)? And how many kids with depression actually go on to be bipolar? One recent paper says half, a significant figure: is it accurate? More research needs to be done, but we do have one longitudinal study that indicated a high rate of remission and relapse with low rates of true "cure."

The Treatment

For bipolar disorder, it is essential to treat the child with a mood stabilizer or an atypical antipsychotic. Mood stabilizers include lithium and the older anticonvulsants Tegretol and Depakote. More recently, the less-tested anticonvulsants Neurontin (gabapentin), Lamictal (lamotrogine), Topamax (topiramate), Gabitril (tiagabine), and Trileptal (oxcarbazepine) have been used in bipolar children.

High doses of these medications are often necessary, which means your child's blood levels should be checked, and she should be watched closely for side effects. You may not see the drug's full effect on the child's mood instability and associated problems until 3 months have passed. If, at that point, the child hasn't responded or hasn't been able to tolerate the drug, the doctor should consider other agents. In some cases—such as when the child does not respond to lithium or an anticonvulsant individually—your child may require two mood-stabilizing agents. I frequently combine Depakote or Trileptal with lithium, as I did with 12-year-old Jay, who is now doing well with 600 mg of Trileptal twice a day and 300 mg of lithium twice a day. In my practice it is common to use a full dose of one medication and a lower dose of the second mood-stabilizing agent.

Over the past few years, clinicians tend to employ the atypical antipsychotics as first-line agents for the treatment of children and adolescents who have severe disruptive disorders, self-injurious behavior, and bipolar disorder. The atypical antipsychotics have been invaluable to assist not only in controlling the manic symptoms (e.g., explosiveness, grandiosity) but also the depressive symptoms of the disorder. The use of atypical antipsychotics for a whole host of disorders in children and adolescents (including tic disorders) is predicated upon a number of studies demonstrating their efficacy for mania and depression in bipolar youth, tic disorders, explosive disorders, and disruptive disorders. In addition, these agents appear to work very quickly, with some trials showing vast changes in behavior already by 2 weeks.

There are also new antipsychotics—Geodon (ziprasidone) and Abilify (aripiprazole)—and we've amassed much more data on risperidone, olanzapine, and quetiapine since this book was first published. And, in addition to Topamax (topiramate), the newer anticonvulsants/mood stabilizer options now include Trileptal (oxcarbazepine).

Antipsychotics should be considered immediately for children with prominent mixed symptoms, acute mania, nonresponse to mood stabilizers, and/or hallucinations. Because the traditional antipsychotics such as Thorazine have disturbing side effects, the newer "atypical" class of antipsychotics is being used: low doses of Zyprexa (olanzapine), Risperdal (risperidone), Seroquel (quetiapine), Geodon (ziprasidone), and Abilify (aripiprazole) are often used in the evening to assist with sleep and reduce the moodiness of the disorder and in the morning for moodiness during the day, with very good success. Unlike the mood stabilizers, the atypical antipsychotics work relatively rapidly—within 2–6 weeks.

When prominent symptoms of depression are part of your child's bipolar disorder, the doctor may prescribe both a mood stabilizer and an antidepressant, but the antidepressant should be short-acting to reduce the risk of severe activation or worsening of mania. The SSRIs (Prozac, Zoloft, Paxil, Luvox, Celexa, Lexapro) are noted for activating mania in bipolar individuals, but Wellbutrin can be introduced gently with less concern about activation. Often agents such as Effexor and Serzone appear to be relatively well tolerated in bipolar youth. Lamictal has recently been FDA-approved for bipolar disorder and is especially effective for the depression. It is not uncommon to use Lamictal to help combat and keep away depression in bipolar kids.

> **activation:** The stimulation of emotional, cognitive, or behavioral processes.

Data show that ADHD responds to treatment *only* if the mood (mania or depression) is being treated. The bipolar symptoms need to be treated *first*. If your child has bipolar disorder and ADHD, a common overlap, the doctor may try an atypical antipsychotic and/or a mood stabilizer for the bipolar disorder and a stimulant—clonidine, Tenex, Wellbutrin, atomoxetine, or a tricyclic antidepressant for the ADHD.

Many young people with bipolar disorder have multiple other problems and do not respond to a single mood-stabilizing agent or antipsychotic. It is not uncommon for these children to receive four different classes of medication. One 10-year-old girl with bipolar disorder, ADHD, and anxiety whom I treat has finally stabilized, after multiple hospitalizations and medication trials, on Trileptal, Zyprexa, Topamax, and Valium. As a parent, you must be sure you are aware of what each agent is targeting and the potential drug interactions among all of them. The Zyprexa and Trileptal are for the mood, the Valium for anxiety, and the Topamax for the weight gain associated with Zyprexa.

Usually, mood stabilizers and/or atypical antipsychotics will need to be continued indefinitely until there is little evidence of mood swings over a period of time. Children and their parents often mistake the long-term effects of these medications for a "cure," and understandably, when the child has been doing so well for a few months, question the need to continue the medication. I strongly recommend that you discuss the matter thoroughly with your child's doctor. Prematurely discontinuing treatment imposes the risk of major relapse and perhaps psychiatric hospitalization (see page 136). If you are leaning in the direction of a trial off the medication, talk to the doctor about trying a very slow taper off one medication at

TABLE 7. Pharmacotherapy of Juvenile Mood Disorders Pharmacotherapy

Disorder	Pharmacotherapy
Depression Major depression Dysthymia	Selective serotonin reuptake inhibitors: Prozac, Zoloft, Paxil, Luvox, Celexa, Lexapro
	Atypical antidepressants: Wellbutrin, Effexor, Serzone, Remeron, duloxetine (may be useful for depression but not FDA-approved as of the writing of this edition)
	Tricyclic antidepressants: imipramine, nortriptyline, desipramine, amitriptyline, clomipramine
	Antidepressants + antipsychotics (e.g., Seroquel) if problems with hallucinations or problems in reality
	Antidepressants + benzodiazepines (e.g., Ativan) if anxiety
	For nonresponders use combined medication strategies: antidepressant + lithium, thyroid hormone, or stimulants
	Electroconvulsive therapy (ECT)
Bipolar disorder (manic–depressive disorder)	Mood stabilizer: lithium (Eskalith, Cibalith, Lithobid)
	Tegretol (carbamazepine) or Trileptal (oxcarbazepine)
	Valproate (Depakote, Depakene sprinkles, valproic acid)
	Other anticonvulsants (Lamictal, Neurontin, Topamax, Gabitril)
	Antipsychotics if psychosis, acute mania, prominent mixed cycles
	Atypical antipsychotics: Risperdal, Zyprexa, Seroquel, Geodon, Abilify
	For nonresponders use lithium and anticonvulsant, or two anticonvulsants
	If agitation or anxiety, add benzodiazepine (e.g., Klonopin)
	If ADHD use Wellbutrin, stimulants, clonidine

a time so you can observe your child's behavior as he safely comes off the medication. Data in adults suggest that rapid discontinuation (less than 1 week) compared to slow discontinuation (1 month) may lead to recurrence of the bipolar disorder and more difficulty treating the disorder in the future. Close communication with your child's school and frequent contact with your child's doctor are paramount during discontinuation phases on mood stabilizers or atypical antipsychotics.

CHAPTER 8

ANXIETY-RELATED DISORDERS

ANXIETY DISORDERS OF CHILDHOOD

These disorders vary widely in how they arise and how they affect children, but they all have one thing in common: ongoing excessive anxiety, worrying, or nervousness. Children with these disorders are not just "worry warts." Their anxiety is exaggerated, inappropriate for their age or developmental level, pervasive, and out of proportion to the situation at hand. It can make the child's daily life a misery. The child not only feels the agony of mental and physical distress but may engineer his entire life to avoid anxiety-provoking situations—all without really understanding what is happening. Needless to say, such machinations can have far-reaching social ramifications. For instance, many children will refuse to go to school, avoid playing with other kids, or be unable to speak in front of even a small group of children.

Childhood anxiety disorders are relatively common, with an estimated 4% of 11-year-olds having separation anxiety disorder and 2% having simple phobia. In 14- to 16-year-olds, 5% have phobias. A phobia is a specific fear that leads to avoidance of situations in which the fear might be triggered, such as not going outside because of a fear of snakes. A simple phobia is a specific fear (and generally avoidance of the thing feared), such as of spiders, heights, or animals.

A growing literature suggests that shyness can be identified in very young children and that it may continue into adolescence and in some cases turn into an anxiety disorder. In many cases, anxiety disorders apparently persist into adulthood. Of interest, many adults being treated for anxiety problems say their disorder began in adolescence.

By their very nature, anxiety symptoms are often internalized. If we add in the shame that many children feel over their "weakness" and "fear," it should be no surprise that many children do not report these problems to their parents. Therefore, it is up to you to be a vigilant observer. If your observations lead you to suspect your child may have anxiety problems, ask her directly if she worries, feels nervous, or sometimes just feels bad for unknown reasons. Here's what to look for, the most common ways that anxiety disorders appear in children and adolescents.

The Disorders

Separation Anxiety

Among the common disorders of childhood, separation anxiety is characterized by excessive anxiety over separation from a caretaker or familiar surroundings. Although some separation anxiety is normal in younger children, when this problem persists, say into the school years, it may prove to be an anxiety disorder. Toddlers, for example, are notorious for forcing their parents to go through absurd gyrations to "sneak out" when leaving the child with a sitter; however, similar behavior in an 8-year-old is problematic.

Obviously the problem can be debilitating to an older child, who may refuse to go to school or develop stomachaches or headaches at school that force the child to return home. These children will often comment that they are afraid something "bad" will happen to their parents or siblings when they are away from home.

Generalized Anxiety Disorder

Michael, age 7, worries incessantly about performing well in school, particularly before a quiz. He had been evaluated by his pediatrician for multiple stomach problems, none of which were found on more extensive testing. In my office, he appeared anxious and reported feeling "funny inside." He noted "worrying all of the time" but said he'd never experienced panic attacks. Michael is typical of children who have generalized anxiety disorder.

Children who are excessively worried about minor matters or schoolwork, are overly concerned about what others think of them, and are perfectionists may have generalized anxiety disorder. These kids often complain about feeling on edge or restless inside. They commonly obsess over upcoming tests or projects. They also usually have multiple physical complaints such as stomachaches, diarrhea, headaches, and muscle tightness and have been seen multiple times in the pediatrician's or school nurse's office for minor medical complaints.

Panic Disorder

Children with panic disorder have attacks of excessive fear for no particular reason. The racing heart and rapid breathing that accompany these attacks often land the child in the pediatrician's or pediatric neurologist's office. These kids may also have "anger attacks" when asked to participate in an event or when they are placed in a situation that makes them feel trapped. When they do, they may lash out at someone who is handy or is instrumental in putting them in the "threatening" situation—often you, the parent.

Agoraphobia is another frequent companion of panic disorder. This fear of going where escape is limited (such as into a car or to school) may move the child to refuse to leave home or may restrict the child's travel greatly. Children may venture out only with a companion. Being unable to get into a car and be driven home from school to play with a friend puts obvious crimps in a child's social life. Fear of buses, trains, and other forms of transportation may require you to arrange for a companion to keep the child calm when he is going somewhere. In some cases, though, the behavior is mystifying and difficult to recognize as agoraphobia. Seven-year-old Zoe, generally soft-spoken and described as "very sweet," would whine and then suddenly lash out at her mother in anger right before they left home to go shopping. It wasn't until her parents found out the same behavior was occurring to a lesser extent on the school bus that they began to suspect something was wrong.

Social Phobia

Among the most common anxiety-based problems to affect children, adolescents, and adults is social phobia, a fear of humiliation in social situations. Socially phobic kids have marked difficulty talking or making a presentation in front of other kids and adults because they are nervous about saying something embarrassing. Although social phobia is generally not treated because in the past it was not thought to be serious or disabling enough to warrant intervention, the condition can be debilitating when severe and can inhibit children from talking in front of their peers even in informal groups. At the least, it can cause kids to miss school on days with scheduled oral presentations or group discussions.

In evaluating your child for an anxiety disorder, it is very important that the doctor look for the possibility of coexisting emotional problems such as depression as well as behavioral problems such as ADHD. Interestingly, children with shyness seem to be at reduced risk for later substance problems, whereas adolescents with an anxiety disorder such as generalized anxiety are at increased risk for a substance use problem. It may be that some of these children are self-medicating their distressing anxiety symptoms.

The Treatment

Both psychotherapy and medication have been shown to be effective for anxiety problems. Behavioral modification and relaxation techniques can reduce anxiety and the resulting avoidance in children. Seven-year-old Michael, for example, gained much improvement in his generalized anxiety disorder with behavioral modification focused on relaxation imagery.

Although there are not a large number of studies in this area, children and adolescents with anxiety disorders appear to respond to the same pharmacological approaches as adult patients. We now have some controlled data on SSRIs (fluvoxamine) for anxiety disorders (first of the kind); hence, SSRIs are first-line now for generalized anxiety, separation anxiety, and panic disorder. Some children will respond favorably in the short term to the sedative, over-the-counter older antihistamines (such as Benadryl or Atarax). Unfortunately, these agents often are overly sedating and work for only a few days. Therefore the pharmacotherapy of anxiety relies on the antidepressants and benzodiazepines (Valium-like medications), often used conjointly with behavioral modification. Seven-year-old Zoe, introduced on page 173, got much relief from the agoraphobia stemming from her panic disorder with behavioral modification plus the brief use of Ativan.

The antidepressants have been used increasingly for anxiety disorders in children, particularly when the anxiety appears chronic (longstanding). The newer antidepressants—Prozac, Luvox, Paxil, Lexapro, Celexa, Effexor, Zoloft, and Serzone—probably are not quite as effective as the benzodiazepines, but they may be an excellent choice if your child has co-occurring depression or obsessive–compulsive disorder. One drawback is that these medications generally need to be used at full antidepressant dosing. To avoid the risk of initial worsening of anxiety or panic, I usually start children on these medications at a very low dose (e.g., Zoloft at 25 mg) and increase them slowly until the parents and I see improvement in the child's anxiety.

If anxiety co-occurs with ADHD, Strattera is probably a good choice. The role of Strattera for anxiety disorders alone is unstudied. The older antidepressants, called the *tricyclics*, including nortriptyline, imipramine, and others, are considered second- or third-line drugs of choice for anxiety. These agents may, however, be a very good choice if your child has anxiety plus ADHD.

For your child, one of the benzodiazepines—Valium (diazepam), Klonopin (clonazepam), Ativan (lorazepam), Serax (oxazepam), Xanax (alprazolam), and Tranxene (clorazepate), to name a few—may be the practitioner's first or second medication choice. Almost any of the anxiety-breaking medications will be useful for a typical anxiety problem. For children with panic disorder in particular, the stronger medications in this class, such as Klonopin, Xanax, or Ativan, are usually prescribed.

The benzodiazepines have been used for many years for a host of problems including seizures and muscle spasms. Because of their effectiveness, excellent margin of safety, and minimal interactions with other drugs, benzodiazepines, along with antihistamines, are also used to treat agitation and insomnia. As a parent you should be aware, though, that these anxiety-breaking agents may produce an opposite reaction in children called *disinhibition* (see page 124). While not dangerous to the child, this paradoxical effect results in restlessness, anxiety, panic, giddiness, and more disturbed behavior, which often starts within 20 minutes of taking the medication. If this reaction should occur, just carefully observe your child and wait it out; the behavior generally subsides within a couple of hours. There is no antidote.

The benzodiazepines can be abused and hence should be supervised closely. While we are not so concerned about your child's developing an addiction to these medications, other kids may approach your child to use his or her medication. These medications generally should be avoided in adolescents with a substance problem.

Of the nonbenzodiazepines, a novel drug called Buspar (buspirone) is also being prescribed for children with anxiety. See page 245 for more details on the drug. If you have reason to seek a medication with little or no abuse potential, you may want to read about and discuss Buspar with your child's doctor.

When kids do have anxiety and another disorder, they often need a combination of agents. I treat a 16-year-old girl with generalized anxiety and obsessive–compulsive disorder who is doing very well on Ativan 1 mg twice daily and 60 mg of Paxil. 1 also treat a 12-year-old boy with panic disorder, ADHD, and depression who, after many failed pharmacological trials, is now stable on 50 mg of nortriptyline at night, 1 mg twice daily of Xanax, and 50 mg of Zoloft with breakfast. The recent introduction of Straterra for ADHD has been an extremely useful addition for youngsters with ADHD and prominent anxiety. I recently treated Kai, an 11-year-old boy with ADHD and generalized anxiety disorder, successfully with 60 mg daily of Strattera. He reported much less anxiety, better attention, and improved quality of life.

Since anxiety disorders are known to wax and wane, periodic tapers to evaluate the continued need for medications are recommended. In some cases children require the medications (or higher doses) only around the beginning (August to November) or end (May to June) of the school year.

POSTTRAUMATIC STRESS DISORDER

The Disorder

Posttraumatic stress disorder (PTSD) is just what its name implies: a combination of ongoing symptoms caused by the stress of having suffered a trauma. A trauma is considered a severe stressor that falls outside the sphere of normal human existence. It may include emotional, physical, or sexual abuse or the witnessing of a calamitous event and may consist of a single incident or repeated exposure to a stressor. Remember, however, that although many children are exposed to trauma, only a small group develop PTSD. PTSD is often accompanied by other psychiatric disorders, including depression and anxiety. The symptoms of the disorder may last less than a month, in which case they are referred to as *acute,* or continue for a long time (*chronic*). The most common symptoms are a physically overaroused state (*hyperarousal*), emotional numbing or callousness, *dissociation* (feeling as if the child is outside of her body), avoidance of situations reminiscent of the event(s), nervousness and excessive startle, and intrusive recollections of the event.

There is a growing consensus in the field that, given the ability of the brain to change during development, severe or repeated trauma in children may result in persistent subtle structural and biochemical changes in the brain. The extent of this process and specific changes have yet to be fully understood, however.

The Treatment

When the trauma suffered is some type of ongoing abuse, the first step in treatment of PTSD is to ensure that the child is in a safe environment. Whatever the trauma, over time, stability in the environment and the child's communication with parents or caregivers are often very helpful in reducing the impairment caused by the PTSD symptoms. Psychotherapy can be invaluable in assisting children in disentangling what occurred and why and in working through many of the issues associated with the trauma, particularly if it continued over a period of time.

No particular medication regimen has been found effective for PTSD, so your child's doctor is likely to target the child's most impairing and persistent symptoms for pharmacological treatment. For example, I found clonidine (0.1 mg) very helpful in reducing not only the sleep disturbance but also the nighttime anxiety of a 7-year-old girl who had been sexually abused and was unable to sleep despite months of counseling. For physically overaroused children who tend to startle easily, antihypertensive agents or a beta blocker such as propanolol can be useful. The antidepressants or the Valium-like medications (benzodiazepines) can help children whose functioning is disrupted by severe avoidance or nervousness.

For those who are plagued by repeated breaks with reality or "out-of-body" experiences (called *dissociative episodes*), techniques such as grounding can reconnect the child to the current environment. Grounding entails, for example, reminding the child where she or he is and what is going on around her or him. If these dissociative episodes are prominent, impairing, or scary to your child, the doctor may also try antipsychotic agents such as Zyprexa or Risperdal at low doses.

Children suffering from posttraumatic stress often have depression and anxiety disorders at the same time. If an evaluation produces such a diagnosis for your child, the practitioner may try an antidepressant such as one of the SSRIs (Prozac, Zoloft, Luvox, Paxil, Celexa, Lexapro), a tricyclic antidepressant (nortriptyline, imipramine, and others), Serzone, Trazodone, Remeron, or other medications. Emotional numbing, however, responds poorly to pharmacological treatment. If your child has several problems related to posttraumatic stress, a combination of agents may be needed. I have used very low doses of Prozac (5 mg a day by suspension) and Catapres (half a tablet twice a day) with excellent response in children with agitation, overarousal, irritability, depression, and sleep disturbances. It is important to remember, however, that many children with multiple PTSD symptoms will overcome them with time, environmental change, and therapy. If your child is among these kids, think of any medication prescribed as temporary treatment, and make sure the child's doctor closely monitors your son or daughter to assess the continued need for it.

OBSESSIVE–COMPULSIVE DISORDER

The Disorder

Obsessive–compulsive disorder has been estimated to affect 1–2% of the population and is believed to begin most often in childhood or adolescence; it is one of the best studied in the family of juvenile anxiety disorders.

Children with obsessive–compulsive disorder are subject to persistent ideas or impulses (*obsessions*) that may lead to repetitive, purposeful behaviors (*compulsions*) that they feel they must complete. Their obsessions are intrusive and senseless and may center on their having caused violence, on sexual perversion, on the need for symmetry, on the danger of becoming contaminated, or on severe self-doubts. Children with obsessive–compulsive disorder may at times appear so severely mentally ill that they have been confused with schizophrenic children.

One less common problem related to obsessive–compulsive disorder is hair pulling (*trichotillomania*). A child who has trichotillomania may pull out her or his hair, eyebrows, or the hair of pets or stuffed animals, to the point of suffering complete hair loss (*alopecia*) that requires a hat to cover. Like obsessive–compulsive disorder, this hair pulling seems to occur more often when the child is not involved in activities.

Most children report being aware of their obsessions and/or compulsions and not liking them. However, when they are prevented from completing the rituals intended to neutralize the obsessive worries, whether these rituals involve handwashing, counting, checking, or touching something, the children become very anxious.

Recent work indicates this syndrome is related to a disturbance in the neurotransmitter serotonin, particularly in the front areas of the brain above the eyes.

The Treatment

Cognitive-behavioral treatment (especially a form called "exposure plus response prevention") is the only effective form of psychotherapy for obsessive–compulsive disorder and is often used conjointly with medications. Within the pharmacological domain, antidepressants that make more serotonin available seem to be the most effective in reducing many of the disabling symptoms of the disorder. This class of medications is well studied, though Anafranil, Zoloft, and Luvox are the only FDA-approved treatments for pediatric patients with obsessive–compulsive disorder. There is also a substantial literature on other antidepressants such as Prozac, Paxil, and Celexa. Studies indicate that relatively higher doses of these medications—300 mg of Luvox in the case of 12-year-old Peter—may be necessary for adequate treatment of juvenile obsessive–compulsive disorder. In more severe or poorly responding cases of obsessive–compulsive disorder, the doctor may need to use Anafranil with an SSRI such as Celexa, an SSRI with a benzodiazepine (like Klonopin), or an SSRI with a low-dose atypical antipsychotic.

If your child has trichotillomania, the practitioner will probably recommend similar medication treatment. Don't expect too much, though. Anecdotal information suggests that the disorder responds only partially to treatment, particularly when the child's trichotillomania begins before puberty.

TABLE 8. Pharmacotherapy of Anxiety-Related Disorders

Disorder	Pharmacotherapy

Generalized anxiety disorder	Antidepressants
	    Selective serotonin reuptake inhibitors: Paxil, Zoloft, Luvox,
	        Celexa, Prozac
	    Atypical antidepressants: Serzone, Remeron

	Anxiety-breaking agents (benzodiazepine): Valium, Tranxene, Ativan, Klonopin, others
	Buspar (buspirone)
	Strattera (atomoxetine)
Panic disorder, separation anxiety	Higher-potency agents: Ativan, Klonopin, Xanax

	Antidepressants
	    Selective serotonin reuptake inhibitors: Paxil, Zoloft, Luvox,
	        Celexa, Prozac
	    Atypical antidepressants: Serzone, Remeron

	Combined pharmacotherapy for nonresponders or children with other disorders (e.g., Tranxene + Prozac, imipramine + Klonopin)
Posttraumatic stress disorder	Treat target symptoms (e.g., anxiety, psychosis)
	Antidepressants: Selective serotonin reuptake inhibitors (e.g., Lexapro), atypical antidepressants, tricyclic antidepressants
	Anxiety-breaking medications: Tranxene, Klonopin, Ativan, others
	If problems with depersonalization or psychosis, consider antipsychotics
Obsessive–compulsive disorder	Selective serotonin reuptake inhibitors: Zoloft, Prozac, Paxil, Luvox, Celexa
	May need higher doses
	Anafranil
	Selective serotonin reuptake inhibitors or Anafranil + benzodiazepine (e.g., Klonopin or Ativan) or Buspar
	Combined pharmacotherapy for nonresponders (e.g., Zoloft + Anafranil or selective serotonin reuptake inhibitor + atypical antipsychotic) or children with other disorders

CHAPTER 9

SCHIZOPHRENIA AND OTHER PSYCHOTIC DISORDERS

THE DISORDERS

Psychosis generally means abnormal thinking that includes substantial problems with reality awareness. In fact, your child should not be diagnosed as psychotic unless the boy or girl has either delusions or hallucinations. *Delusions* are false, implausible beliefs. *Hallucinations* are false perceptions involving any of the senses—visual (sight), auditory (hearing), tactile (touch), or olfactory (smell). Many psychotic children have both. Eight-year-old Karin, for example, described hearing voices "outside of her head" (hallucinations) and also was convinced that someone was poisoning her food (delusion).

As in adults, psychotic disorders in children are categorized as functional or organic. Functional psychoses are mental illnesses, including schizophrenia, schizoaffective disorder, and severe forms of mood disorders in which the child suffers breaks in reality. Organic psychosis refers to damage to the brain or central nervous system as a result of medical illness, trauma, or drug use.

In children with either type of psychosis, imaging tests may show that certain areas of the brain are slightly smaller than in nonpsychotic children. Neuropsychological testing often shows profound abnormalities in a child's ability to ascertain, perceive, manipulate, store, and recall information. In many cases, the brain's processing problem occurs far in advance of the breaks in reality.

Although the causes of schizophrenia are not well defined, congenital (birth) brain malformations and genetics are among the most likely contributors.

For parents the challenge is recognizing that a serious problem exists, requiring a full evaluation. Children are notorious for not telling their parents about their hallucinations or delusions. It is not unusual for me to find out during an evaluation that a child has been hearing voices for 2 years and has not told anybody. Often children don't know that the voices talking to them are abnormal or are afraid to tell others about them. When a psychosis begins or worsens, however, the child is likely to display severe behavioral problems, including having outbursts, acting strangely, or withdrawing. These types of behavior should certainly signal you to investigate, and in fact that is why children are usually brought to me.

Psychotic disorders in children often start insidiously and may follow other preexisting problems. Children who develop psychotic disorders may have early symptoms of other psychiatric and neurological disorders. Some children start out with ADHD-like symptoms (see page 143), which progress in intensity and level of disorganization. In other children you may notice a "flat" mood, which is often followed by the onset of hallucinations. Yet others may feel mild weakness in an arm or leg and then begin to behave in bizarre ways. Most children develop these uncharacteristic behaviors, often along with hallucinations (usually auditory). Unfortunately, these disorders typically continue through childhood, often getting worse as the child gets older.

THE TREATMENT

Antipsychotic drugs, also referred to as *major tranquilizers* or *neuroleptics,* are the standard treatment for psychotic disorders in children. Your child's doctor may prescribe any of a large number of medications, including Haldol, Thorazine, Trilafon, Stelazine, and others. Be aware, however, that these medications cannot resolve all problems that accompany psychosis. The target problems or symptoms that most commonly respond to antipsychotics are the so-called *positive symptoms*—active problems such as hallucinations, delusions, formal thought disorder (incoherence), and/or catatonic symptoms (stupor, negativism, rigidity, and posturing) or bizarre feeling states. In contrast, the *negative symptoms*—important elements that are missing from the child's emotional makeup—are not as likely to be improved by the older antipsychotics. Because of unresolved lack of emotionality, little speech and thought, lack of involvement in activities (*apathy*), inability to enjoy (*anhedonia*), and poor social functioning, many psychotic children continue to have ongoing difficulties with day-to-day life.

The newer antipsychotics, Risperdal, Zyprexa, Seroquel, Geodon, and Abilify, appear to be more effective for treating negative symptoms and for treating the more active positive symptoms with fewer side effects. Therefore, when an evaluation uncovers a picture that suggests long-standing psychotic symptoms, such as those that indicate schizophrenia, many practitioners now start the child on Risperdal, Zyprexa, or Seroquel. Clozaril is reserved for children who do not respond to multiple trials of older and newer antipsychotics.

Because antipsychotic medications are often used with other agents, it is important to be aware that they generally increase the blood levels of the other medications, such as increasing nortriptyline levels by 30%. Likewise, certain antidepressants (Prozac and others) increase the effectiveness of the antipsychotics.

Parents can take comfort in the fact that children with psychotic problems such as schizophrenia have been helped greatly by our improved understanding of the disorder and the new generation of medications available for their treatment. Though you can expect your child's problems to continue into adulthood, providing the child with the new medications and a low-stress, structured environment should allow your son or daughter some normalcy in childhood and hope for the future.

TABLE 9. Pharmacotherapy of Schizophrenia and Psychotic Disorders

---

Atypical antipsychotics: Risperdal, Zyprexa, Abilify, Seroquel, Geodon
  May be tried as first-line drugs of choice
  Clozaril reserved for children not responding to treatment

Standard antipsychotics: Trilafon, Haldol, Thorazine, Stelazine
  Caution with risk for tardive dyskinesia

For agitation, add high-potency benzodiazepines (e.g., Ativan, Klonopin, Xanax)

For children not responding to treatment
  Use atypical antipsychotic
  Switch antipsychotic class: from Thorazine to Trilafon, from Navane to Zyprexa
  Combine treatments

If mood swings present, antipsychotics + lithium, mood-stabilizing anticonvulsants
  If severe outbursts, antipsychotics + propanolol
  If marked anxiety, antipsychotics + benzodiazepines (i.e., Klonopin, Ativan)

CHAPTER 10

DISORDERS OF KNOWN MEDICAL AND NEUROLOGICAL ORIGIN

TICS AND TOURETTE'S DISORDER

Despite the fact that they are clearly medical or neurological in nature, a number of childhood behavioral problems end up being diagnosed and treated by mental health professionals. This happens in part because the major symptoms are psychiatric—rage, for example—and in part because certain psychiatric symptoms or disorders tend to co-occur (OCD and ADHD, for instance, commonly appear with Tourette's disorder). Because psychotropic medications are commonly used to treat both the major symptoms of the disorders discussed in this chapter and the co-occurring psychiatric disturbances, it makes sense to consult a mental health practitioner for your child.

The Disorders

Tics are relatively common in children, with surveys indicating that approximately 15% of children will have them at some point. They range from the twitches and spasms known as *motor tics* to the verbal noises called *phonic tics.* Tics can also be *simple,* such as a twitch, or *complex,* including bending, grimacing, or shrugging.

Children whose tics last longer than 1 year are considered to have chronic tic disorders. We simply do not know why some tics last and some do not. We do know, however, that at least 50% of the tics that begin in childhood disappear by age 18.

If your child has not only motor tics but also phonic (verbal) tics and other behavioral and psychological symptoms, the child's diagnosis will be Tourette's disorder. The child's phonic or vocal tics usually show up as coughing or throat clearing, but they may appear in the form that has gotten the most publicity: the shouting of swear words (*copralalia*). The phonic tics that Tourette's features have caused much misunderstanding about the disorder because at times they appear to be and may be willful.

Tourette's disorder begins in childhood and sometimes lasts throughout life. Its symptoms often fluctuate spontaneously over time. Stressors, such as starting the school year or simply discussing the child's tics, often accentuate them by raising the child's level of anxiety. Although children may have some ability to suppress their tics temporarily when they are specifically directed to do so, they usually have little long-term control over them.

Complicating the picture, it is not uncommon for disturbing behavioral patterns to surface, based to some degree on comorbid disorders. In fact, you and your child's doctor will have to make treatment decisions on the understanding that in many cases these co-occurring disorders, not the primary tic or Tourette's disorder, are the major source of distress and disability. A growing research effort has been directed at unraveling the connections between tic/Tourette's disorders and the disorders with which they often co-occur—anxiety disorders, obsessive–compulsive disorder, and ADHD: How are they related? Is any cause and effect involved? What genes cause tics or Tourette's disorder, and why do these tics often get turned on and off spontaneously?

Much of this interest has been aimed at the overlap of tic and Tourette's disorders with obsessive–compulsive disorder. Studies at Yale University have uncovered two interesting interrelations:

1. About one-third of the children with Tourette's disorder have significant obsessive–compulsive symptoms.
2. A sizable number of children with severe tics or Tourette's disorder have a relative with obsessive–compulsive disorder, leading researchers to believe that these two disorders are genetically connected.

Similarly, interesting associations with ADHD have been identified in other research:

1. Approximately half of children with Tourette's disorder have ADHD.
2. ADHD appears earlier in life than tics.
3. Many of the behavioral problems and impairment in these children are related to the ADHD.
4. The use of stimulants may or may not worsen tics.

The Treatment

Behavioral modification can be very useful in diminishing many of the aberrant behaviors that may emerge or in helping children fight their complex tics, such as repetitive writhing, standing up and turning around, and touching body parts in a specific manner. Cognitive-behavioral therapy may help the child identify when these behaviors are occurring, what sets them off, and how the child can "relax" herself and, to some degree, control these repetitive acts. Pharmacological approaches to tics and Tourette's disorder have evolved greatly over the past two decades. Unfortunately, because the order and availability of medications for tics and Tourette's have changed so dramatically over that decade, many practitioners are not up to date on the current treatments.

The antihypertensives clonidine and, to a lesser extent, Tenex have become the first line of treatment for tics and Tourette's disorder. They work quite well—two-thirds of children respond favorably—but you can expect an accurate evaluation of their effectiveness in your child to take 2–4 weeks. The necessary dose varies greatly, so the doctor will probably start your child on a low dosage and increase it depending on response and side effects.

The tricyclic antidepressants—desipramine, nortriptyline, imipramine, amitriptyline—have also been found useful in controlling tics and Tourette's disorder. As with the hypertensives, dosing should be started low and increased up to typical "full" dosing based on side effects and response. Both classes of drugs are particularly helpful for the large group of children with concurrent Tourette's disorder and ADHD.

When more conventional treatments fail to help children with Tourette's disorder, the antipsychotic drugs, particularly Haldol and Orap, are the medications of choice. Despite their good treatment record, however, antipsychotics have a couple of significant drawbacks: They have limited effects on the frequently associated disorders such as obsessive–compulsive disorder; and they carry significant risk for the development of both short- and long-term adverse effects, one of the most feared being tardive dyskinesia (see page 259). For these reasons, you should make

TABLE 10. Pharmacotherapy of Tics and Tourette's Disorder

Clonidine (Catapres)

Tenex (guanfacine)

Tricyclic antidepressants: desipramine, imipramine, nortriptyline

Klonopin (clonazepam)

High-potency antipsychotics: Risperdal, Haldol, Orap, Prolixin, Geodon, Abilify

Strattera

Combined pharmacotherapy for treatment nonresponders or children with other disorders: clonidine plus Zoloft, desipramine plus Concerta (watch for possible tic worsening with stimulants), clonidine plus Ritalin LA

sure other pharmacological interventions are tried first. More recently, clinicians are using the newest generation of antipsychotics, including Risperdal, Geodon, Abilify, and Zyprexa, since they appear to have fewer short- and long-term side effects than the older antipsychotics such as Haldol and Orap. Children who also have obsessive–compulsive disorder may need additional pharmacotherapy with serotonergic drugs such as Anafranil or the SSRIs such as Luvox or Prozac (which alone have little effect on tics). Children with ADHD plus tics may need a medicine for the tics like clonidine and one for the ADHD like a stimulant. Strattera has also demonstrated improvement in tics in children with ADHD and tics.

> **serotonergic:** Related to serotonin, the chemical messenger in the nervous system related to mood, anxiety, aggression, and sleep.

TEMPORAL LOBE EPILEPSY (TLE), COMPLEX PARTIAL SEIZURES

The Disorder

Juan, age 15, was admitted to a psychiatric hospital for irritability, hypochondriasis, and "bizarre thoughts." On examination, he was found to have multiple hallucinations—distortions, bizarre smells and tastes—as well as unreal perceptions such as the feeling of having been somewhere (*déjà vu*) and the feeling of being outside of his body (*depersonalization*).

Eighteen-year-old Dominick had been hospitalized four times, all for severe rage attacks. Both have a type of seizure disorder called *complex partial seizures,* or *temporal lobe epilepsy (TLE).* Unlike the grand mal seizures that we think of when epilepsy is mentioned, temporal lobe epilepsy does not make children shake and lose consciousness. Instead, it causes emotional and behavioral disturbances in the form of periodic, heightened states such as marked moodiness or rage, leading to outbursts for no apparent reason. The disorder appears in children of all ages. These disturbances are caused by seizures, or abnormal electrical activity in the brain. The seizures occur deep in the brain substance located at about the level of the ears, in the region called the *temporal lobes.* This region of the brain is related to emotion, perception, and memory, and seizures here affect the major communication lines within the brain. Consequently, children with this type of seizure may report variable psychic symptoms. Many of them involve perceptual distortions. Visually they might include seeing objects as bigger or smaller than they are or seeing shadows in the periphery, or side, of their visual fields. These distortions can also affect the senses of smell and taste; children report abnormal smells such as burning tires and metallic tastes. Feelings of (*déjà vu*) are related to disturbances in memory. These somewhat bizarre experiences can occur steadily or wax and wane.

> **psychic:** Related to a wide array of perceptual and emotional states, such as heightened emotions or rage.

TLE is not a common disorder and is not easy to diagnose. Only a thorough history that turns up the types of symptoms just described is likely to lead an evaluator in the right direction. Once TLE is suspected, an electroencephalogram (EEG) should be completed to look for abnormal brain electrical activity. To help elicit seizure activity, the EEG may need to be completed both while the child is awake and while he or she is asleep. This type of EEG is called a *sleep–awake EEG* and generally requires keeping your child awake all night, or at least awakening the child after he or she has slept only from midnight until 3:00 A.M. If your child has to undergo a sleep–awake EEG, be prepared for the "fun and excitement" of forcing him or her to remain awake while terribly sleepy.

In Juan's case, a sleep-awake EEG indicated abnormal seizure activity in the temporal lobes and led to pharmacological treatment. In Dominick's case, the EEG was normal, but a 24-hour EEG, in which the patient wears the EEG monitor for a day while going about his normal routine, revealed periodic seizure activity on the left side of the brain in the temporal lobe. These seizures coincided with the marked anger attacks Dominick recorded in a diary.

In cases of an abnormal EEG, some children are asked to have a brain imaging scan. Whereas the EEG may identify abnormal electrical activity in the brain, brain imaging tests—CT or MRI—can uncover problems with the brain substance itself (tumors, birth malformations, artery problems, etc.).

The Treatment

Medications for children with temporal lobe epilepsy include the older anti-convulsant medications Tegretol (carbamazepine) and Depakote (valproic acid) and the newer agents Trileptal (oxcarbazepine), Neurontin (gabapentin), and Lamictal (lamotrigine). These seizures commonly require higher doses of the anticonvulsant agents, which means the blood levels of some of the medications in the child must be monitored closely. Juan's symptoms were markedly improved with Tegretol, and in Dominick's case the same drug eliminated his rage attacks altogether.

If your child does not respond to a single agent, two anticonvulsants may be necessary. If the child has hallucinations, the doctor may want to add an antipsychotic medication to the anticonvulsants. The anxiety-breaking medications (benzodiazepines) such as Klonopin (clonazepam) may be helpful if your child has prominent anxiety. Interestingly, Klonopin has been used at higher doses of 6–12 mg daily for seizures and in fact is FDA-approved for use as an anticonvulsant in children.

As with other seizure disorders, the doctor should reassess your child periodically and should discontinue medication if the child's symptoms are gone and the child's EEG is normal. Most often, TLE continues into adulthood, which means your child will need ongoing anticonvulsant treatment. Dominick's treatment continues to be effective 5 years after he began taking Tegretol.

ORGANIC MENTAL DISORDERS AND BRAIN INJURY

The Disorder

Sadly, a significant number of children suffer some sort of brain damage that causes emotional or behavioral disorders. Generally these problems are called *mental disorders due to medical conditions*. These disorders can be congenital, which means they occur at birth for no apparent reason, they can be caused by *in utero* trauma (such as fetal distress), or they can be caused by birth trauma. At any later point in the child's life, they can be caused by encephalitis (infection of the brain), meningitis (infection of the lining of the brain), toxicity (drugs or exposure to harmful agents), or blunt trauma such as a bicycle or motor vehicle accident.

Children with brain injury are known to exhibit a wide array of behaviors such as disinhibition (acting out of control, being exceedingly silly, or overreacting), rage attacks, temper tantrums, aggression, panic reactions, and isolation or withdrawal.

The Treatment

How these children are treated depends on the specific symptoms or problems the child has. The more common symptoms are the externalizing or acting-out problems, and for these, behavioral modification should be tried first. This form of therapy may be very helpful in reducing specific symptoms. Medications found helpful for aggression and acting out include the mood stabilizers (lithium, Tegretol, Depakote), Valium-like medications (benzodiazepines such as Klonopin), antihypertensives (propranolol, guanfacine, clonidine), antipsychotics (Thorazine, Zyprexa, and others), and Trexane or Rivea (naltrexone). If there are prominent symptoms of inattention/distractibility, impulsivity, and/or hyperactivity, medications for ADHD may be tried. For severe cases, especially those in which children are harmful to themselves or others, multiple medications may need to be prescribed. Plan to keep a diary documenting outbursts and other "target" behaviors during medication trials.

CHAPTER 11

OTHER MENTAL HEALTH DISTURBANCES AFFECTING CHILDREN AND ADOLESCENTS

EATING DISORDERS: ANOREXIA AND BULIMIA

The Disorders

Anorexia nervosa (commonly called *anorexia)* and bulimia nervosa (commonly called *bulimia)* are both complicated eating disorders that affect mainly girls and young women, although some boys and older men and women suffer from the disorder as well.

Anorexia is defined by profound weight loss or the inability to maintain a body weight higher than 15% below the "ideal body weight" (the suggested weight for the height and age of the child). People with anorexia report feeling and looking fat, even though to others they often appear frail or very thin. Anorexic girls often to do not begin to have their menstrual periods or lose their periods *(amenorrhea)* during their episodes of decreased eating. These children and adolescents are obsessed with issues surrounding food and may exercise excessively.

Bulimia is characterized by repeated episodes of overeating (bingeing), often intermixed with attempts to vomit (purge), abuse laxatives, or exercise excessively. Bulimic young people, usually girls, are preoccupied with weight, as are anorexics, but unlike anorexics they do not necessarily feel or perceive that they are overweight. In fact, most bulimics range from normal weight to slightly overweight. Often stress and feelings of hopelessness or depression will worsen the bulimia.

In both anorexia and bulimia, co-occurring disorders are very common. Depression, anxiety, PTSD, and personality issues often accompany the eating disorders, and it is possible to see traits of both anorexia and bulimia simultaneously in the same child. Although the neurobiological connection is not well worked out to date, children with eating disorders appear to have disturbances in the brain neurochemicals serotonin and dopamine and in the opioid (*pain control*) system.

Although it is most likely to occur in adolescence, it is not uncommon to see anorexia in children as young as 7 years old and into adult life. The prognosis for anorexics and bulimics is mixed. Although the treatment of anorexia has improved, a child's obsessiveness about food and distorted body image often continue to some degree into adulthood. Progress in treating girls with anorexia is slow, and even children who succeed in gaining weight customarily report feeling uncomfortable and distressed and require encouragement and counseling. Bulimia appears to have a better outcome over time than anorexia. As they grow into young adulthood, many bulimics will harbor the urge to binge or purge during stress but will not act on their urges.

The Treatment

Nonpharmacological treatments for anorexia include a multifaceted approach: family and individual psychotherapy as well as nutritional counseling. These are often very helpful in identifying family and individual dynamic issues as well as educating the family about the often long-standing condition. Various members of your family, including your child, other children, and you and your significant other, may very well require therapy.

The SSRI antidepressants (Prozac, Zoloft, Celexa, Luvox, and Paxil) have been shown to be somewhat effective and may be worth trying. These antidepressants may help primarily by reducing the anorectic's urges, craving, and obsessions, but they sometimes cause the unwelcome side effect of actually increasing weight loss. If an antidepressant is prescribed for your child, be vigilant in watching for further weight loss.

Identification and treatment of co-occurring disorders such as anxiety or depression may hold out hope for improving an anorexic child's condition and quality of life. For children with severe anxiety, the benzodiazepines (Valium-like medications) may be beneficial. Rarely, children with anorexia may require antipsychotics because of their profound distortions in thought.

For bulimia, nonmedication treatments are similar to those used for anorexia. As with anorexia, therapy and medications are often combined, although bulimic teenagers may respond better to medications than anorectics. The tricyclic antidepressants (desipramine, imipramine, amitriptyline) and the SSRIs (Zoloft, Prozac, Luvox, Celexa, and Paxil) are often helpful in reducing the binge-and-purge cycles. For children with prominent mood swings, the doctor may prescribe lithium, Depakote, Trileptal, Neurontin, or other mood stabilizers.

Recently, sibitramine (Meridia) and Topamax have been shown to be effective in reducing binge eating (sibitramine) and purging (Topamax) in bulimic subjects and is worthy of consideration. Sally is a 17-year-old senior who reported binging and purging daily for 1 year. She had a history of depression that was not currently problematic. Psychotherapy plus Topamax at 100 mg daily was very effective in helping her stop her bulimia.

ALCOHOL AND SUBSTANCE ABUSE

The Disorder

Many adolescents and, to a lesser extent, children have tried alcohol and/or drugs sometime during their lives. Studies indicate that over half of high school seniors have used alcohol and marijuana, and approximately 25% have smoked cigarettes. A smaller group of approximately 10–15% have used cocaine, amphetamines, and inhalants. What makes a child start using cigarettes, other drugs, or alcohol is not entirely known. Availability, community and personal values, level of self-esteem, peer pressure, parental substance use, and a host of other issues appear related. In addition, studies indicate that a family history of alcoholism or drug abuse puts children at substantial risk for substance abuse. A well-known study based in Sweden indicated a ninefold risk for alcoholism in the sons of fathers with alcoholism. Other studies have shown that juvenile-onset substance abuse runs in families, is highly inheritable, and is often accompanied by conduct (delinquency) and mood disorders. In fact it is now clear that approximately three-quarters of adolescents with substance abuse also have a psychiatric disorder (comorbidity) and that psychiatric disorders untreated result in higher risk for cigarette smoking and substance abuse.

Determining the difference among normal use, misuse, and abuse or dependency can be difficult. *Use* generally means infrequent to occasional use of a substance commonly used by others in the community with little direct harm to the adolescent. *Misuse* indicates a pattern of use with some consequences of the substance use. *Abuse* and *dependence* are more serious disorders in which the child has begun to lose control of the substance ("needs to get high"). Alcohol or drug abuse is diagnosed when there is an established and often continued pattern of substance use despite legal, interpersonal, or medical consequences. Direct evidence of abuse includes blackouts, substance use prior to or during school, substance use alone or with strangers, driving while intoxicated, and consumption in dangerous situations. Changes in school or work performance, fights, irritability, and a lack of interest in activities or motivation are indirect evidence that your child may be involved in substance abuse.

Dependence is usually presumed by a mental health practitioner when the child demonstrates a daily pattern of excess substance use for which there are more serious consequences such as school failure or legal problems. Dependent adolescents may become physiologically addicted and may have difficulty stopping their substance or alcohol use because of disturbing withdrawal symptoms or psychological dependence. Cigarette use is one of the most common substance use problems in adolescents in general and in those with psychiatric disorders in particular. Young people who smoke tend to have higher rates of mental health problems, and conversely, higher rates of cigarette use tend to be seen in psychiatrically impaired juveniles. It is important to mention your child's nicotine use (including chewing tobacco) to the doctor not only to address the child's addiction but also because of the potential for drug interactions—nicotine can increase or decrease the amount of the prescribed medication in the child's system.

The psychiatric conditions most often seen with substance problems in children are conduct disorder, ADHD, oppositional defiant disorder, depression, bipolar disorder, and to a lesser extent anxiety and panic disorders. In many cases the psychiatric problem precedes the substance problem, leading to conjecture that many children "self-medicate" their symptoms by using substances. In addition, children with psychiatric problems may not have the foresight or inhibition it takes to resist getting involved with alcohol or drugs. This appears to be the case with ADHD. The myth that taking stimulant medications for ADHD leads to later substance abuse persists to this day, even though it seems more and more certain that it is the impulsivity of ADHD that often leads these kids to use alcohol or illegal drugs. In January 2003 I published a paper (in the journal *Pediatrics*) that reanalyzed the world's literature on stimulants and substance abuse, finding that treatment of ADHD *reduces* the risk for substance abuse by half.

The Treatment

There is no unifying treatment for alcohol or drug problems. Initially, both you and your child need to understand what substances are being misused and what risks that misuse brings. Following that, it is important that you take several measures:

- Monitor your children to deter further use. Random urine toxic screens to detect illicit substances in your child's body provided by the child's practitioner or school can be useful. When teens complain that requiring drug tests demonstrates a lack of trust in them, I find it helpful to comment that it is "the disorder of addiction" that is distrusted, not necessarily the child. For kids who refuse or are unable to leave a urine sample for analysis, hair testing or saliva testing is now available.
- Provide additional structure yourself or arrange for it to be provided by your child's school and afterschool programs.
- Look into support groups such as Alateen, Alcoholics or Narcotics Anonymous, and Rational Recovery for teens and their families.
- Seek appropriate psychotherapy. Research indicates that family therapy, behavioral modification, and coping skills training (how to deal with life stressors) are the most effective types of psychotherapeutic intervention for adolescent substance abusers.
- For cigarette use, apply the same cessation techniques that adults use and also reduce your child's access to cigarettes. Use of the nicotine patch or nicotine gum in concert with Zyban (bupropion) can be highly effective in helping an adolescent stop smoking cigarettes or using snuff.

The pharmacotherapy that your child's doctor devises will be aimed at reducing the child's craving and diminishing the child's underlying psychiatric disturbance. Medications that reduce cravings include those used to replace the dangerous street drugs (and accompanying high-risk behavior). Methadone, for example, is a synthetic and long-acting narcotic agent that supplants the need to obtain and use heroin every few hours. More recently, the SSRIs and Wellbutrin have been used in adults with limited effectiveness for reducing drug cravings. Naltrexone has also been shown useful in reducing alcohol consumption in adult alcoholics but remains un-studied in teens. Similarly, Wellbutrin and nicotine patch es/gum have been shown effective in cigarette cessation in adults but have only limited data in children and adolescents.

Most pharmacotherapy in adolescents with substance use disorders is aimed at the underlying or co-occurring disorders, such as ADHD, which occurs in about one-quarter of the teenagers with a significant drug or alcohol habit, and depression, which occurs in about half of them. It's not always clear, however, whether these other conditions are primary or secondary disorders. Depression, for example, can just as easily be a prod-uct of substance abuse and will disappear once the child has been sober or abstinent for a certain period of time.

Often, then, your child's doctor may wait until the child has been so-ber for 1–4 months before diagnosing or initiating medication treatment for a majority of disorders. For some conditions such as bipolar disorder or schizophrenia, it may be necessary to start medication before the child stops abusing the substance. Studies show that treating a substance-abus-ing adolescent with bipolar disorder with lithium reduces the substance abuse. If your child has developed a substance problem while on medica-tion, most doctors will not restart the medication until the child has been "clean" for 1 month. Make sure your child gets the message directly and clearly from the doctor: *No substance abuse while taking prescribed medica-tion.*

Beyond that caveat, the timing of treatments is done on a case-by-case basis and depends on a thorough evaluation of the child's functioning with family, peers, and school. Elena had been using LSD and marijuana daily, and I suspected that her depression had been a cause—not a re-sult—of her substance abuse because of what else I learned about her: She had "fallen in with the wrong crowd" recently, and though her school performance was low, it had not always been that way. After she had suc-cessfully stopped using drugs for 4 months, Elena continued to appear de-pressed, with low energy and sadness, and so she was treated with a very low dose (25 mg per day) of a new antidepressant, Effexor. Her mood im-proved, she reunited with her old friends, and she has been performing well academically for the last year with no substance use.

There are no special rules for treating underlying psychiatric prob-lems in cases of substance abuse, though we have more established algo-rithms for treating adolescents with substance abuse and other disorders. For example, one should treat bipolar disorder in a substance-abusing ad-olescent with bipolar disorder. Such is probably the case for depression (now not seen to be entirely secondary to the effect of substances of abuse on the brain). ADHD is a mixed bag, the recent consensus being to stabilize the addiction and then treat the ADHD relatively rapidly. As for anxiety/obsessive–compulsive disorder, doctors typically recommend behavioral treatments, then SSRIs.

Your child's practitioner may take one of these approaches:

- Young people with ADHD benefit from the traditional regimens, including Wellbutrin, the tricyclic antidepressants, the antihypertensives, and the extended-release stimulants. Should kids who have a recent history of drug or alcohol problems be placed on the stimulants? This is a common concern, but since these medications are the best studied and most effective agents for ADHD, their use in "high-risk" groups is acceptable as long as the children are monitored closely. Your child's doctor might consider initially using a stimulant with a lower abuse potential such as Cylert, followed by Concerta, Metadate CD, or Ritalin LA and then by the extended-release amphetamine compounds (Adderall XR) or Dexedrine spansules.
- Co-occurring juvenile depressive disorders are best treated with antidepressants, including the SSRIs (Prozac, Zoloft, Paxil, Celexa, Lexapro, and Luvox), Wellbutrin, Remeron, Serzone or Trazodone, Effexor, and less commonly the tricyclic antidepressants (nortriptyline, imipramine, and others).
- Children with bipolar disorder will require atypical antipsychotics and/or mood stabilizers, which should be started as soon as the diagnosis is made—even if the adolescent is still abusing drugs or alcohol—as mentioned above.
- Adolescents with a history of substance abuse in whom anxiety is a problem can be tried on nonaddictive anxiety-breaking compounds such as Buspar, the SSRI or tricyclic antidepressants, Serzone, Remeron, Effexor, and more distantly the Valium-like benzodiazepines.

To ensure your child's safety, frequent discussions with your child's practitioner are paramount. Adequate monitoring by you, the doctor, and other caregivers is necessary to make sure that your teen is not using substances, to evaluate the effectiveness of the medication, to check compliance, and to assess for potential drug interactions. Although most medications are safe when combined with periodic alcohol or drug use, the literature has included a number of cases in which children developed delirium, severe blackouts, agitation, and medical complications after mixing them with street drugs. For example, our group recently reported that using marijuana while taking nortriptyline or desipramine caused severe delirium in a number of patients. While not studied systematically, there appears to be good relative safety of the combined use of the stimulants (methylphenidate and amphetamine-based compounds), Wellbutrin, Strattera, mood stabilizers, and atypical antipsychotics with the major substances of abuse: alcohol and marijuana.

If you suspect your child is using a particular drug while receiving a prescribed psychotropic, in addition to your child's physician you may wish to contact the U.S. Poison Control Centers for information about potential drug interactions and suggested instructions.

SLEEP DISTURBANCES

The Disorders

Sleep disturbances are common in children, and it is perfectly normal for them to occur temporarily during certain developmental stages. They are, however, often reported by parents whose children have psychiatric disorders. Sleep disorders may also lead to behavioral and cognitive symptoms that could be construed as psychiatric in nature.

Some disturbances that affect sleep itself appear to be related to the mental disorder, such as a reduction in sleep related to a depression or a manic episode in a bipolar child. Another group that often has these sleep disturbances are children with ADHD. Although this is not well documented in laboratory sleep studies, reports from parents indicate that ADHD children have difficulty falling asleep, sleep poorly, and have difficulty awakening. Children with sleep apnea or prominent snoring may be at increased risk for behavioral problems. Conversely, some children with depression may oversleep both at night and during the day.

Other disturbances involve abnormal behavior or events during sleep—nightmares, sleep terrors, sleepwalking, and sleeptalking. These disturbances occur during various sleeping states and may be related both to the underlying psychiatric disorder and to its treatment. Children with mood disorders may report violent, scary dreams. The use of certain medications such as tricyclic antidepressants and clonidine may produce nightmares; however, few medications are related to sleepwalking.

The Treatment

Correction of the underlying psychiatric disorder can assist in reducing a sleep problem. For example, 16-year-old Sam, who has bipolar disorder, says his first sign of becoming manic is a change in his sleep cycle. Whereas Sam usually sleeps for 8 hours, when feeling manic symptoms, he sleeps for only 3–4 hours and feels fully rested. In these cases the lithium is increased, and often his antipsychotic agent (Mellaril) is restarted at night.

Evaluation of the nature of the sleep disturbance is the first step. Nonpharmacological treatments should be tried initially in children with sleep difficulties. Structure and routine are of great help: eliminate caffeinated beverages (certain colas, tea, hot chocolate), reduce activity around bedtime, and try playing soft music or relaxation tapes to help your child go to sleep easily. Make sure your child avoids strenuous activity prior to bedtime. Whereas some children find the computer relaxing, others become stimulated by it and should avoid contact with the computer prior to bedtime. Awaken children early and avoid letting them take daytime naps. One 8-year-old patient of mine with ADHD was in the habit of going to bed at 9:00 P.M. but would not fall asleep until midnight; then he would nap for up to 2 hours every day after school. After about 2 weeks of keeping him from napping (no small task!), his parents saw his sleep cycle return to normal.

Medications for sleep problems should not be used without careful thought and a hypothesis about what is causing or exacerbating the sleep problem. Over-the-counter medications such as antihistamines (Benadryl, Dimetapp, and others) may be useful on an as-needed basis for passing sleep problems. Dosages ranging from half a teaspoon (12.5 mg) to 1 teaspoon (25 mg) in a child or 2 teaspoons (50 mg) in an adolescent are generally effective. Although usually quite safe, they may cause excessive morning sedation and dry mouth, and the child often becomes tolerant of the medication's sleep-producing effects.

Clonidine is a commonly prescribed agent for sleep, particularly if the sleep problem is related to ADHD or other psychiatric disorders. Generally it is started at half a tablet (0.05 mg) and increased as necessary, which should be supervised by your doctor. In our clinic, we recently reported on a study in which children received Catapres safely for up to 3 years, with the majority of parents reporting an excellent continued response.

Other agents include the Valium-like medications such as Ambien, Klonopin, or Ativan. These medications may cause marked daytime sedation, disinhibition, and nightmares and are generally not used over the long haul. In addition, they should be avoided in cases of substance abuse since they may be addictive, although there are few data to indicate a problem with everyday use in juveniles.

Melatonin has been reported to be useful in controlled studies in adults and by a number of parents of children in our clinic. Although it is essentially untested for safety, efficacy, or proper dosing, most children seem to respond favorably to lower dosing (0.5 mg at night). Like other *soporifics* (sleep-inducing agents), melatonin may cause morning sedation. Sedating antidepressants such as amitriptyline or imipramine (25–75 mg) or Remeron (7.5–15 mg) can be useful not only for promoting sleep but also to help treat bedwetting, ADHD, and anxiety.

Some children develop a sleep problem only in response to their medication. Most notable are the stimulants, which are notorious for producing insomnia (difficulty in sleeping). In those cases, earlier administration of the medication or a reduction in the dose may alleviate the problem. If the daytime medication is very effective and needs to be given, another medication at bedtime may be beneficial. Bedtime doses of clonidine, melatonin, Remeron, and amitriptyline have been reported to be useful in stimulant-induced sleep problems associated with ADHD.

For children who have severe recalcitrant sleep problems or sleep problems related to psychotic disorders (bipolar disorder or schizophrenic illness), the antipsychotics may be necessary. Most commonly, Thorazine, Mellaril, Zyprexa, or Risperdal is used and may cause confusion, heaviness, excess sedation, and abnormal muscle movements. Since long-term use may cause irreversible involuntary muscle movements (tardive dyskinesia), especially with the older agents (Thorazine, Mellaril), this class of medications should not be used unless other treatments have not proven successful or if psychosis is present.

ENURESIS

Bedwetting (*enuresis*) in children is not uncommon, with up to 15% of 11-year-old boys still having difficulties with this problem. There is often a family history of bedwetting, generally in the father. Bedwetting is thought to represent an immature neurological system and not the presence of major mental illness. Bedwetting without a known medical cause such as infection usually responds to nonpharmacological therapies such as behavior modification. A number of commercial products that take a behavioral approach to reducing nighttime bedwetting are available.

Pharmacological treatment relies on two very different agents: a synthetic hormone or a tricyclic antidepressant. With both agents, relief is generally immediate, but discontinuation will lead to return of the bedwetting. The nose spray, whose agent is now available in a tablet, antidiuretic hormone desmopressin (ddAVP), has been shown to be effective for the treatment of bedwetting, although it is expensive. It is relatively free from side effects except occasional irritation of the inside lining (mucosa) of the child's nostrils when used in nasal spray form. Imipramine and other tricyclic antidepressants at doses of 25–50 mg nightly have also been shown to be effective.

Trials off medication should be attempted periodically since enuresis may remit spontaneously. Medications may also be used intermittently when the child is involved in sleepovers and overnight camps where the embarrassment of bedwetting may be significant.

PART III

The Psychotropic
Medications

This section presents detailed information on the medications referred to in Parts I and II—how the medications work, which disorders they are used to treat, typical dosage ranges and other information on administering the drug, and side effects to watch for. Charts will sum up important facts and provide a handy cross-reference of brand (marketed name) and generic (chemical) names for each drug. The section moves from most to least commonly prescribed drugs for psychiatric problems in children.

Questions that parents ask time and again in my office reveal that there is much confusion over the terms used to categorize and name these drugs: "How can a drug called a stimulant be right for my hyperactive son?" "Why would you prescribe an antidepressant for my daughter when we both agree she's not suffering from depression?" "Can you explain—in English—what a selective serotonin reuptake inhibitor is?" "Why do they call some antipsychotics atypical?" These are all valid questions. Medications with psychoactive properties used to treat behavioral and emotional difficulties in children and teenagers are globally referred to as *psychotropics*, but beyond that the terminology becomes quite confusing.

Most of the compounds you are about to read about are classified generally by their effectiveness in treating adult disorders—antidepressants for depression, antihypertensives for high blood pressure, antipsychotics for psychosis, mood stabilizers for mood disorders, and anxiolytics for anxiety. Others are named for the effect they have on behavior—the mood stabilizers, for example—or for their similarities to other compounds, as in the case of the stimulants. More specific medications are named for their chemical structures (tricyclic antidepressants) or how they work in the brain (selective serotonin reuptake inhibitors).

To complicate matters further, a number of medications are considered one type of compound but are used for another problem. For example, clonidine and Tenex are antihypertensives—that is, they lower blood pressure—but are used in psychiatry to treat tics and ADHD. While the tricyclic antidepressants are commonly used for ADHD, enuresis (bedwetting), and anxiety, they are rarely used for depression these days in youth.

Why use these labels to head the following chapters if they are so misleading? First, because realistically they are what you will encounter in discussions with all mental health professionals. Even more important, though, understanding these classifications will help you become an informed collaborator in your child's care. In today's health care atmosphere, it's quite likely that your child will have different doctors over the years. The more you understand about your child's medication history—"No, John was constantly giddy on Ativan, so I'd be worried about trying Klonopin" or "Yes, we'd be willing to try Prozac, but you should know that Zoloft didn't help"—the more you can preserve continuity of care for your child. Keeping track of each drug's classification on your medication log (see page 115) might help you maintain a clear picture of your child's course of treatment.

Don't let the chemical structures, mechanisms, or names of the medications intimidate you—just remember to write down the names of the medication (brand and generic) that your child will be taking, and when you have *any* question about a medication being prescribed for your child, ask the prescriber, the pharmacist, and anyone else who is participating in the care of your child.

CHAPTER 12

THE STIMULANTS
AND NONSTIMULANTS FOR ADHD

You may already know more about the stimulant medications than any other drugs used to treat psychiatric disorders in children. Not only are they the most commonly used and well-studied psychotropic agents in children and adolescents today, but they have received a lot of attention in the popular press.

The stimulants have been around since their usefulness was described in 1937 in the United States, and today over one million children in this country alone are being treated with these medications. That figure represents a substantial increase over the last decade, which can be traced to increased identification and treatment of ADHD, particularly in those with the inattentive form, in girls, in adults, and in people with other psychiatric disorders. The number of people requiring treatment has grown even further now that families and mental health practitioners are recognizing that ADHD often persists beyond adolescence and into adulthood.

Perhaps because of their increasing visibility, the stimulants continue to be under the scrutiny—and sometimes under the fire—of the media. Reports ranging from stunting of growth to stimulation of aggression have left many parents hesitant to authorize stimulant treatment of their children with ADHD. As a parent making important health decisions for your child, you should know that much of the hype about aggression originated in individual cases rather than in broad cross-sections of young patients.

In a number of those cases, the teenagers involved had not been taking the stimulants within a year of the incidents reported, so there is no cause-and-effect link.

If you decide on a trial of stimulants for your child, the medications the prescriber is most likely to name are methylphenidate (Ritalin, Ritalin LA, Metadate, Concerta), dextroamphetamine (Dexedrine, Adderall), and pemoline (Cylert). Except for Cylert, the stimulants are under strict control by the Drug Enforcement Administration and are classified as schedule II. This means you will have to be prepared to get monthly or bimonthly rewritten prescriptions and to provide a picture ID at the pharmacy. Cylert, too, is carefully monitored, but physicians may call the prescription in to the pharmacy and also renew it rather than write a new prescription. Of note, various mail-order prescription services allow a 3-month supply of a stimulant. Contact your insurance carrier to see if it provides such a service.

HOW THE STIMULANTS WORK

The stimulant medications, while they are in a child's blood system, appear to normalize biochemistry in the parts of the brain involved in ADHD. Specifically, they enhance nerve-to-nerve communication by making more neurotransmitters available to boost the "signal" between neurons. The stimulants work by blocking the recycle mechanism of the sending nerve cell, leading to an accumulation of the neurotransmitter, which is then available to pass on the signal. The neurotransmitters that are released more effectively when a child takes stimulants are dopamine and norepinephrine.

You may wonder why, if they all enhance nerve-to-nerve communication, there is such a selection of stimulants for the doctor to choose from. The fact is that each class (methylphenidate vs. amphetamine) may have a slightly different mechanism of action. This means that, despite their similarities, different stimulants may reduce your child's ADHD symptoms to different degrees. Don't be discouraged, then, if a trial of Ritalin or Concerta has disappointing results in your child; he may respond very well to Dexedrine, Adderall XR, or Cylert instead. Be patient and be prepared for some experimentation—strategies to try when your child does not respond to a medication are in Table 11.

All told, the stimulants are effective in approximately three-quarters of those with ADHD—children, adolescents, and adults included. The

DRUG ENFORCEMENT AGENCY (DEA) DRUG SCHEDULING

The Drug Enforcement Administration "schedules" a drug based largely on its abuse potential (*liability*), either by the individual taking the medication or by others who may steal the medication, diverting it from its proper use. Prescribed medications that are watched very carefully and require special prescribing practices are considered *schedule II*. Among more frequently prescribed psychotropic medications, schedule II compounds include Ritalin, Concerta, Metadate, Dexedrine, and Adderall. Different federal, state, and local laws govern the use of schedule II compounds, but generally prescriptions for them must be issued either monthly or bimonthly and patients have only 3–5 days to fill the prescriptions.

Thought to be less likely to be abused, schedule IV compounds are prescribed medications that are also watched carefully but allow for refills and more latitude in the time allotted to fill the prescription. Schedule IV compounds include Cylert, the benzodiazepines (Valium, Klonopin, Ativan, Tranxene, others), and narcotic painkillers (such as Percocet).

Because the laws applying to both schedule II and schedule IV drugs come from several levels of government, how pharmacies handle these prescriptions varies from location to location. For example, some pharmacies will allow a 2-month prescription of Ritalin, whereas others allow for only 1 month's supply. Likewise, some pharmacies require two forms of identification to fill a prescription, whereas others need only one. Try to remain patient with the rules and feel free to ask the pharmacist about any laws and regulations he or she is obligated to follow in filling your child's prescription. On the other hand, alert your child's doctor if you feel the pharmacy is being punitive or overly restrictive in allowing you access to prescribed medications.

stimulants are among the best-studied medications in medicine, with their safety and effectiveness in ADHD assessed in well over 250 controlled studies of more than 5,000 patients. This research has demonstrated that the stimulants can diminish the inattention, distractibility, overactivity, and impulsivity that disrupt the lives of ADHD children and adults. Likewise, stimulants have been shown effective in improving child–mother interactions, peer relationships, academic performance, and classroom behavior. Both research and clinical experience indicate that boys and

TABLE 11. What to Do If Your Child Does Not Respond to the Stimulant Medications*

Symptoms	Intervention
Worsened or unchanged ADHD symptoms (impulsivity, hyperactivity, inattention, distractibility)	• Increase stimulant dose. • Change timing of administration. • Change preparation (extended to short-acting). • Substitute stimulant (Ritalin to Dexedrine). • Consider alternative treatment (Strattera, antidepressant, clonidine).

Intolerable side effects	• Assess if side effect is drug-induced.
	• Determine when side effect is occurring (peak vs. wearoff).
	• Consider changing
	  1. Timing of dose (give earlier or later in day)
	  2. Preparation (e.g., short-acting to extended-release)
	  3. Type of stimulant (e.g., Dexedrine to Metadate CD)
	  4. Manufacturer (generic to brand)
	• Use adjunctive medication (e.g., clonidine, Remeron, for sleep).

Marked rebound	• Change preparation to an extended-release form. • Change timing of administration. • Add another small dosing 30 minutes prior to rebound symptoms (e.g., 2.5 mg of Focalin). • Consider alternative treatment. • Consider adjunctive Strattera or tricyclic antidepressant or clonidine in afternoon.
Development of, or use with, tics or Tourette's disorder	• Assess continuation of tics off stimulant. • If tics stop, try stimulant again. • If tics continue, discontinue stimulants. • Use alternative treatment (Strattera, clonidine, tricyclic antidepressants). • If ADHD symptoms continue, cautiously reintroduce stimulant. • Consider use with adjunctive treatment (Strattera, clonidine, desipramine, Risperdal, Geodon, Haldol, Orap).

(cont.)

TABLE 11. *(cont.)*

Symptoms	Intervention
Emergence of marked sadness, anxiety, agitation, irritability	• Assess timing for toxicity (at peak effect 1–2 hours after taking) or withdrawal (during the rebound or wearoff phase, 6–12 hours later). • Reduce or change dosing. • Evaluate for return of ADHD symptoms. • Evaluate for another psychiatric disorder. • Change preparations or substitute type (Adderall to Concerta). • Discontinue stimulants. • Consider alternative treatment (Strattera, antidepressant).

*In each case, determine if the stimulant is helpful. If there has been no response, reevaluate the dose and consider trying either another form of the stimulant or, if tried, another type of medication.

girls get equal benefits from the stimulants, as do people of all ages, from preschool through adulthood.

One recent study of ADHD without other psychiatric or learning disabilities showed that the stimulants not only can have long-term benefits but also may be sufficient treatment on their own. After 2 years of follow-up, Ritalin was still very effective in reducing the core ADHD symptoms, and additional multimodal treatment (parent training and psychotherapy) did not add substantially to the medication's already significant effect. You and your child's doctor will want to consider this fact if your child responds well to medication—additional psychotherapy is not automatically warranted.

THE PRESCRIPTION

The most commonly prescribed and best-known stimulant is methylphenidate. All of the brand-name stimulants but Cylert—Ritalin, Dexedrine, and the amphetamine compounds (Adderall)—have preparations that are on the shorter-acting end of the spectrum. They all have approximately the same efficacy (see Table 12). You'll probably see the medication's effect on your child's attentiveness and behavior within 30–60 minutes after the child takes it (once a correct dose is reached via the process described

How can a stimulant possibly make my son less active?

I can see why you would be skeptical, and many parents are—we all think of stimulants as drugs that keep us awake and aroused. The low to moderate oral doses used to treat ADHD actually make most people—whether they have ADHD or not—more attentive, less distractible, and less active. Those with ADHD get much more "improvement" in these areas than those without ADHD, probably because of the biochemical differences between the two groups.

Can't we try Adderall with my daughter to find out for sure if she has ADHD?

When a child's problems elude diagnosis, it is tempting to use a "proven" treatment to come up with answers. As in all of medicine, though, a response or lack of response to a treatment cannot be relied on to diagnose ADHD. Remember, one-quarter of those with ADHD do not respond to stimulants anyway, so not responding to a stimulant (what the doctor may describe as *"treatment refractory")* does not necessarily mean the child does not have ADHD—and vice versa.

My daughter was diagnosed with ADHD 7 years ago, and she still needs medication. At first it was all pretty simple (if not easy); Ritalin was pretty much the drug of choice. Now so many different new medicines are available—how do I know which one would be best for her now?

It may be confusing to know what is similar and what is different among all the medications for ADHD on the market today, especially if your child's doctor isn't scrupulously up to date. While Concerta, Metadate CD, and Ritalin LA are all methylphenidate, Adderall XR is amphetamine. Metadate CD and Ritalin LA work for about 8 hours, while Concerta and Adderall XR work for up to 12 hours. See Table 12 for comparisons among them all. Then, in consultation with your child's doctor, determine which advantages are most desirable for your child's health care needs and lifestyle.

TABLE 12. The Preparation and Strength of the Stimulants

Medication			Duration of
Generic name	Brand name	Sizes and preparation	action/form
Methylphenidate	Ritalin	5, 10, 20 mg; tablets	4 hours/tablet
	Ritalin LA	20, 30, 40 mg; capsules	8 hours/capsule
	Focalin	2.5, 5, 10 mg; tablets	5 hours/tablet
	Concerta	18, 27, 36, 54 mg; capsules	12 hours/capsule
	Metadate CD	10, 20 mg; capsules	8 hours/capsule
	Methylin	20 mg; tablets	4 hours/tablet
Dextroamphetamine	Dexedrine	5, 10 mg; tablets	4 hours/tablet or spansule
		5, 10, 15 mg; spansules	
Magnesium pemoline	Cylert	18.75, 37.5, 75 mg; tablets	10 hours/tablet
Amphetamine compounds	Adderall	5, 10, 20, 30 mg; tablets	6 hours/tablet
	Adderall XR	5, 10, 15, 20, 25 30 mg; capsules	12 hours/capsule

on page 113). These effects usually peak between 1 and 4 hours after the drug is taken. This relatively short "behavioral half-life" naturally requires multiple doses to sustain the child's response over the waking hours. Many parents opt for longer-acting or extended-release stimulants so their child does not have to go to the school nurse for a dose of the stimulant. Slow-release preparations usually have a peak clinical effect 30 minutes to 6–8 hours after administration, meaning one dose given in the morning may last the whole school day. Be aware that although 10 mg of Dexedrine is roughly equivalent to 10 mg of the short-acting tablet, 20 mg of sustained-release Ritalin is roughly equivalent to 10 mg of regular Ritalin stretched out through the day. Similarly, 10 mg of methylphenidate given three times daily is equivalent to Concerta 36 mg. To further complicate matters, amphetamine (Dexedrine and Adderall) is about twice as potent as methylphenidate, so 20 mg of methylphenidate is equivalent to 10 mg of amphetamine.

The best solution for stimulant timing problems may be to mix preparations (such as short-acting and sustained-release Ritalin), but arriving at the appropriate combination demands collaboration and communication. As a parent, you need to get feedback on how your child is doing at various points in the school day and then pass on that information to the prescribing doctor. The parents of 7-year-old Ken, for example, knew that their son had severe behavioral difficulties on the school bus and both behavioral and attentional problems in school. The bus drivers and teachers were able to tell them that the 10 mg of short-acting Ritalin Ken was taking helped his school bus ride and earlier hours in school, but the driver and teachers all noted a marked deterioration around noon until 2:00 P.M., as well as on the return bus ride. Together Ken's parents and practitioner decided on a change to the 20-mg sustained-release Ritalin and agreed to watch him closesly. Ken's parents reported to the doctor that the new prescription helped Ken considerably in the later hours at school and on the bus ride home but left him without medication effect in the earlier hours. This time around, they tried a combination of 5-mg regular and 20-mg sustained-release Ritalin, which gave Ken consistent improvements throughout the school day. Most children are now being prescribed the new extended-release preparations of methylphenidate (Concerta, Ritalin LA, Metadate CD) or amphetamine (Adderall XR), which provide sustained treatment of ADHD throughout the school day.

With the increasing interest in treating ADHD throughout the entire day, extended-release preparations of stimulants (Concerta, Ritalin LA, Metadate CD, Adderall XR) are the preferred stimulants of choice. Ritalin, Dexedrine, and Adderall, in contrast, may be given only at the times or in the situations when the symptoms of ADHD cause the child the greatest problems. Parents often consider the school hours the crucial times for medication. But before you choose to withhold medication after school, you should review the problems ADHD may be causing outside school. When medication is withheld, any interpersonal, family, and peer problems caused by ADHD may continue to plague your child during his or her free time. Also, many kids find that difficulty concentrating affects the sports in which they participate; continuing their medication after school greatly benefits their athletic performance and enjoyment. Even sporadic events like long car rides may be easier for your child with the medication's help. In the final analysis, whether to administer stimulants continuously on evenings, weekends, and holidays is an individual decision that should be based on how severely and persuasively your child's social and family life is impaired.

What's the best way to find out how the stimulants are working at school?

As described on pages 113–121, asking a favorite teacher or guidance counselor to give you weekly feedback about your child's behavior and attention will not only provide you with invaluable information but also engage the school system in your child's care. Although some practitioners find the use of teacher report forms helpful in dissecting treatment effects, our group prefers frequent parent contact with the school during the medication initiation phase.

That decision can also be based on what you observe in your child when medication is initiated. The exact nature of positive effects and side effects that your child experiences may help you decide not only whether to give the medication continuously but also how to schedule the doses. If, for example, the appetite suppressant effects of the stimulants are a problem for your child, it may be a good idea to administer the medicine during or after meals. Giving stimulants with food does not appreciably alter your child's body's ability to absorb the medication properly.

To arrive at the proper dose, the prescriber will start with a low dose and gradually increase it until positive effects are observed by you and the child's teachers or until developing side effects signal that a higher dose would be harmful. The starting dose for the short-acting stimulants (Ritalin and Dexedrine) is generally 2.5–5 mg per day and for extended-release 10–20 mg given in the morning and increased with the smallest increment every few days. If prominent wearoff is occurring midday, most prescribers should suggest switching to an extended-release stimulant. Shelly is a 12-year-old girl with ADHD who is doing well on Adderall XR, receiving 20 mg in the morning. Her 8-year-old brother receives 36 mg of Concerta in the morning and sometimes a 5-mg dose of Ritalin in the late afternoon. The wide array of literature on the stimulants also suggests that, in some cases, more medicine may be better than less medicine for controlling both the attentional and behavioral ramifications of ADHD.

---

blood level: The amount or concentration of medication in the blood. Synonymous with *serum* or *plasma concentration.*

My son says he hates to take his medicine, and he has several reasons for feeling this way: He doesn't like to swallow pills, he hates having to go to the school nurse for his midday dose, and he doesn't want to think of himself as being "different." How can I make this easier for him when I know (and he does too) how much better he does on the medication?

The field has been aware of the problems your son has had; new forms of medication are now available that should make your lives easier. Today there are osmotic-release capsules (in which water from the intestine slowly enters the capsule chamber, causing the medication to be "pushed" out a laser-drilled hole in the capsule) and high-tech beaded technology (allowing you to sprinkle the medication on food for kids who have problems taking medications—e.g., Adderall XR and Ritalin LA). There is also a patch (Methypatch) in development, and there are dissolving tablets that don't need to be swallowed. Ask your doctor and pharmacist about the availability of your child's medication in these new forms.

SIDE EFFECTS OF STIMULANTS

You can expect your child to experience some side effects while taking stimulants, but the most common ones often can be managed. Table 13 lists these side effects and what you can do about them. While your child is beginning a trial of stimulants, start a medication log, as described on page xxx, and record the details of the effects you observe. Don't forget to note when these problems are occurring. The timing of side effects can give your child's doctor important clues to what might be causing the effects and how the treatment should be altered. Side effects that occur 1–2 hours after taking the medication are likely related to the peak effect of the medication, whereas those that occur 4–8 hours after your child takes the medication may relate to wearoff from the stimulants (such as tiredness).

The most commonly reported short-term side effects of the stimulants are appetite suppression, sleep disturbances, headaches, and stomachaches. Sadness or irritability as well as worsening of the ADHD during wearoff (called *rebound phenomena*) also appear, but less frequently.

Sleep disturbances can be marked and may diminish the daytime effectiveness of these medications. If your child is having sleep problems on

TABLE 13. Some Management Strategies for Common Stimulant-Related Side Effects

Side effect	Management
Loss of appetite (anorexia), weight loss	• Monitor weight closely. • Give stimulant with meals. • Add calorie-enhanced snacks (ice cream). • Don't force meals. • If sudden onset with Cylert, check liver blood test.
Difficulty falling asleep (insomnia)	• Administer stimulants earlier in day. • Change to shorter-acting forms. • Discontinue afternoon or evening dosing. • Use low-dose clonidine, Benadryl, periactin, Remeron, amitriptyline, or melatonin at bedtime.
Dizziness	• Have your child's blood pressure checked. • Have your child drink more fluids. • Change to extended-release form (Adderall XR, Ritalin LA, Concerta, Adderall).
Rebound phenomena	• Change to extended-release form. • Overlap stimulant dosing (usually by 30 minutes). • Combine long- and short-acting forms. • Use additional treatment (low-dose clonidine or tricyclic antidepressants).

Irritability, sadness, moodiness, agitation	• Evaluate when it occurs.
	    Peak (may be too much medication)
	    Wearoff (see "Rebound" above)
	• Reduce dose.
	• Change to another preparation.
	• Assess for another problem such as depression.
	• Use adjunctive treatment (antidepressants, lithium, anticonvulsants).

Growth problems	• Monitor. • Compare with parental height history. • Attempt weekend and vacation holidays. • Refer to pediatrician. • Change to nonstimulant treatment (Strattera, nortriptyline, clonidine, Tenex, Wellbutrin).

the stimulants, earlier timing of the stimulant, a reduced dose, or a change from a long- to a short-acting form may be necessary. On the other hand, if the child is responding quite well to the stimulant, the doctor may suggest adding a low dose of another medication—clonidine, Remeron, or imipramine—instead. Parents of children who take melatonin to help them sleep have reported no drug interactions with the stimulants.

Irritability or sadness occurring 1–2 hours after dosing may indicate too much medication. Bill had a good response to Dexedrine tablets but had mood symptoms 1 hour after taking each dose. He did very well by simply switching to Adderall. Irritability 4–12 hours after dosing may signal withdrawal. Rebound phenomena can occur in some children between doses, creating uneven and often disturbing symptoms. The good news is that the advent of the extended-release stimulants has virtually eliminated problems with wear-off or rebound. The overlapping of doses or a change to longer-acting preparations may help reduce both withdrawal symptoms and rebound phenomena. Treatment with 10 mg of Ritalin twice a day improved 12-year-old Sally's academic performance and behavior significantly, but her mother reported that Sally was isolating herself when she got home from school and acting "depressed and angry." Sally's afternoon problems went away when we changed her to Concerta. Another strategy could have been to add 2.5 mg or 5 mg of the Ritalin or Focalin when she got home from school to "smooth out" the wearoff from the Ritalin.

Less frequent side effects of the stimulants in children include headaches, repeated movements (such as picking the nails or skin), dizziness, staring spells, stomachaches, and fatigue. Stimulant-associated hallucinations are extremely rare and often signal too high a dose or another underlying problem—notify your child's doctor immediately if this should occur.

Children taking Cylert should have a baseline blood test to see how their liver is functioning before beginning the medication and then at least every 3–6 months or whenever they develop severe flulike symptoms. Cylert has rarely been associated with liver problems (hepatitis) that are generally mild but can be serious. There is no need for blood tests or other physical monitoring other than height and weight measurements with the other stimulants.

For information on drug interactions with the stimulants, see Table 14. Although I do not advocate that adolescents use drugs of abuse when treated for their ADHD, some recent results from controlled clinical trials are comforting in indicating a lack of severe drug reactions reported between stimulants and marijuana, alcohol, or other drugs of abuse.

TABLE 14. Potential Drug Interactions of Stimulants with Commonly Used Drugs

Medication	Comments

Decongestants
  Pseudoephedrine
  (Actifed, Sudafed)
  (Cocaine)
	Can increase both medications' effects; start with lower doses of decongestant.

Antihistamines (Benadryl, Dimetapp)	May diminish effectiveness of stimulants.
Strattera	No noted interaction.
Tricyclic antidepressants	May increase both medications' effects; check blood level of antidepressant.
Anticonvulsants	May increase or decrease anticonvulsant level.
Prozac and related antidepressants; Wellbutrin, Trazodone, Serzone	No noted interaction.
Antibiotics	No noted interaction.
Antipsychotics, anxiety-breaking agents	No noted interaction.

When Disorders Overlap

Some concerns linger over whether the stimulants caused or worsened tic disorders (involuntary muscle spasms) and seizures. Since both of these problems coexist with ADHD in a substantial number of children, you would be wise to keep current with developments on these fronts.

Many professionals now feel that stimulants merely bring out a vulnerability for underlying tics but don't often cause them outright. In part this theory is based on the excess overlap of tics and ADHD: half of children with tics or Tourette's disorder have ADHD, and 15% of ADHD children have tics unrelated to the stimulant treatment or the ADHD. A cautious approach for children with ADHD and tics would be to try nonstimulant treatments such as clonidine, tricyclic antidepressants, or atomoxetine first. Then, if nothing else works for the ADHD, stimulants can be used as long as the child is observed closely for worsening of the tics. If any worsening occurs, immediately take the child off the stimulant medication to see if the stimulants were a direct cause of the worsening.

My own clinical experience agrees with the recent studies that suggest some children with tics can still benefit from stimulants as long as they are monitored carefully. You may read in the *PDR* that stimulants should not be used if your child has a seizure disorder because the stimulant might increase the frequency of seizures. This issue is of utmost importance since a number of children with seizures also have ADHD. Despite what you may read, however, scientific investigations of both absolute seizure rates and brain wave recordings (EEGs) in stimulant-treated children simply do not support this contention. You should also know that many pediatric neurologists use stimulants in children with seizure disorders without reports of worsened seizures. Generally children should be treated for both disorders, which means prescribing stimulants for the ADHD and the appropriate anticonvulsant agents (such as Dilantin, Lamictal, Depakote, Tegretol, or other) for the seizures.

The Effects of Long-Term Stimulant Use

Questions about whether children taking stimulants over long periods suffer impairments in height and weight growth have been asked for the past 2 decades. Unfortunately, this subject is still shrouded in myth, and embarrassingly few data are available. While early and uncontrolled reports prematurely alarmed parents, the most recent information suggests that the vast majority of these children ultimately achieve normal height and weight as young adults. *By nature of their ADHD,* these children tend to mature and grow at a later stage (usually later adolescence) of their life. In other words, they tend to be shorter as children but catch up as adolescents and young adults.

Additionally, the most recent data derived from large multisite studies seem to indicate that stimulants may have a very subtle effect on both weight and height. Children tend not to gain weight over the first 6–9 months of treatment with the stimulants (and Strattera, coincidentally). Over 2 years, data are indicating that children weigh about 3–5 pounds less and may be 0.1–0.5 inches shorter compared to the "normal growth chart" from the Centers for Disease Control and Prevention. Of significance, those children who are already short and thin demonstrate essentially no effect of treatment, whereas those who are the largest and heaviest display the most effect. It may be that extended-release methylphenidate preparations lead to less effect on growth than multiply dosed short-acting agents or amphetamine—this clearly requires further study.

There *is* a small group of ADHD children with a definitive reduction in weight and growth that is attributable to stimulants, but it occurs when the children stop eating, lose weight, and therefore simply do not grow. As a parent, you should keep tabs on your child's growth while he or she is taking any medication. If your child is taking stimulants, watch for a substantial decrease in appetite or a weight loss and take the following precautions:

1. Make sure your child's doctor does a before-treatment assessment and takes height and weight measurements three or four times a year. Your child's height and weight can be charted on growth charts that you can access online at the American Academy of Pediatrics website (*www.aap.org*) or purchase, or that may be available from your child's practitioner.
2. If a decrease in weight is noted during the early phase of treatment, caloric supplements or foods rich in calories (all of the food you don't dare consume!) may be helpful in counteracting the daytime appetite suppression. Data from recent studies with Adderall XR and Concerta indicate that it is common to see a transient effect on weight (i.e., no gain) over the first 6–9 months of treatment followed by resumption of normal weight gain.
3. If stimulant-induced delays or reduction in growth are noticed, talk to the doctor about drug holidays. Studies have demonstrated that stimulant-related effects on growth may be lessened by these periods off the medication. Drug holidays need to be tempered by the sometimes negative effect of medication discontinuation (i.e., untreated ADHD).
4. However, if the height and weight growth problems are severe, they may require switching your child to an alternative treatment. We have found, for instance, that children often gain weight when placed on nortriptyline for their ADHD.

Despite the stimulants' many years of use, we still have no systematically obtained information to disentangle the ways in which medication for ADHD prevents or causes impairment much later in life. The consensus of the field continues to be that assertive treatment of any disorder will result in lessening of the impairment caused by not treating the disorder over time. An example of this is the previously mentioned study that demonstrated significant reductions in substance abuse in ADHD youth previously treated with stimulants.

STRATTERA (ATOMOXETINE)

The first nonstimulant medication for ADHD, Strattera (atomoxetine), was approved relatively recently for the treatment of ADHD in children, adolescents, and adults. Strattera has been studied extensively not only in the use of ADHD itself but also in ADHD plus other psychiatric conditions. As of this printing, there are more than 10 controlled studies including children, adolescents, and adults for ADHD itself demonstrating Straterra to be very useful in the treatment of ADHD. Many studies of Strattera in specific ADHD groups are under way.

Strattera is mechanistically more similar to the older tricyclic antidepressants. Strattera is a highly specific presynaptic (sending neuron) noradrenergic reuptake inhibitor. Strattera makes more norepinephrine (and dopamine) available for nerve-to-nerve communication. Unlike the stimulants, Strattera has absolutely no abuse potential and is not a scheduled medication. Your child's doctor can write prescriptions with renewals and can call this medication in for your child.

Strattera is among first-line agents for ADHD. Because it is relatively new on the market, some doctors are reluctant to initiate treatment with it—instead, they choose to use it for kids who have side effects or incomplete response to stimulants. Studies completed also indicate that it is useful in youth who do not respond to stimulant medications and in those who are intolerant to the adverse effects of stimulants. Strattera has been demonstrated to be helpful in all subtypes of ADHD.

One of the most intriguing applications of Strattera is for the child who has the common co-occurrence of anxiety, tics, or depression with ADHD. Studies show that Strattera is helpful not only in treating the ADHD under these circumstances but also in improving the anxiety, tics, or depression. Strattera has also been useful in reducing the prominent oppositional symptoms often occurring in kids with ADHD. Since Strattera is free of abuse liability (and presumed diversion to other kids), it is an ideal candidate for adolescents who are using substances of abuse. No serious side effects have arisen in conjunction with alcohol or marijuana.

Strattera is readily absorbed in the gastrointestinal tract and peaks in the serum soon after administration. Results from dose-ranging studies indicate an optimal dose based on the weight of the child: 1.2 mg per kg per day, which can be increased to a maximum of 1.8 mg per kg per day. Don't be in a hurry to go to full dosing too rapidly—we have found that it may lead to sedation that is not a problem when starting the medication slowly. In children and adolescents (weighing less than 70 kg), Strattera should be initiated at a total daily dose of 0.5 mg per kg (around 25 mg) and increased after 2 weeks to 1.2 mg per kg per day. In older children and adults, it should be started at 40 mg and increased after 2 weeks to 80 mg and then ultimately to a maximum of 100 mg in those who have not had a maximal effect. Strattera can be given either once or twice daily with similar efficacy and tolerability. I typically start Strattera at night and after 2 weeks convert it to morning administration. Continued efficacy has been reported in the evening even after once-daily administration of Strattera in the morning. No blood monitoring of Strattera levels or other blood tests are necessary.

Strattera is broken down (metabolized) in the liver (hepatic system). While Strattera is generally easy to use, there are potential drug-to-drug interactions, so you should ask your child's doctor before starting other medications. Likewise, if your child is on Strattera, remind the doctor of the potential for a drug interaction.

Strattera is generally well tolerated. Short-term side effects of excessive tiredness (especially when first started—it gets better), insomnia, stomachaches, headaches, nausea, vomiting, and weight loss/appetite suppression have been reported. Strattera also has mild effects on elevating blood pressure and pulse but does not require routine monitoring in youth. However, adults receiving Strattera should have their blood pressure/pulse monitored at baseline and on the drug. Longer-term data suggest continued effectiveness and tolerability of Strattera. It does not escape height and weight concerns. Similar to stimulants, participants on Strattera experienced transient lack of weight gain over the first 6 months. At 2 years, there were continued minor effects on reducing weight, and essentially no major effects on height. As with the stimulants, those individuals who were the smallest and lightest had no effects, whereas those who were heavy and tall had more effects. No serious problems have arisen with its use.

PROVIGIL

Provigil (modafinil) is not a stimulant medication but a wake-promoting agent—a medication that is FDA-approved for narcolepsy. Large trials of Provigil for ADHD have produced mixed results. One large multisite study in children demonstrated a moderate response for the medication, at approximately 200 mg in the morning and 100 mg in the afternoon, in reducing ADHD symptoms with minimal side effects (most commonly headaches, stomachaches, edginess, insomnia). Provigil may be helpful, in my experience, for kids with ADHD who do not respond to more standard medications.

CHOLINESTERASE INHIBITORS

We are currently experimenting with the use of a class of medications used and FDA-approved in adults with Alzheimer's disease called the cholinesterase inhibitors. These medications include Aricept (donepezil), Reminyl (galantamine), and Exelon (rivastigmine). For the most part, these medications work by blocking the enzymes involved in the breakdown of an important neurochemical in the brain, acetylcholine, making more acetylcholine available. Acetylcholine is involved in memory and executive functioning. These medications seem to improve mildly the executive functioning problems (organization, time management, prioritization) that kids with a host of psychiatric disorders may have. Currently, we are using these medications as add-ons (adjunctive) to other medications for ADHD and other disorders. The medications have *not* been systematically safety-tested in youth, and we really do not know about long-term effects; therefore, they should be used judiciously. Short-term side effects include nausea, diarrhea, and dizziness.

CHAPTER 13

THE ANTIDEPRESSANTS

The antidepressants are a wide, diverse group of medications so called because they are all used to treat adults with depression. In children, they also have different benefits: They have been shown scientifically to help children and adolescents with ADHD, obsessive–compulsive disorder, tic disorders, and bedwetting (enuresis). Ironically, the effectiveness of certain antidepressants in children with depression is not as clear.

The main classes of antidepressants are the SSRIs; the atypical antidepressants such as Wellbutrin, Effexor, Remeron, and trazodone; the tricyclic antidepressants; and the MAOIs, which are rarely used in children. The table below lists these medications, and the text in this chapter describes each group separately.

THE SEROTONIN REUPTAKE INHIBITORS

The most commonly used antidepressants for children are called the *selective serotonin reuptake inhibitors,* or SSRIs. These include Prozac (fluoxetine), Paxil (paroxetine), Celexa (citalopram), Zoloft (sertraline), Lexapro (escitalopram), and Luvox (fluvoxamine). Many parents are hesitant to use these widely publicized medications, especially Prozac, because of claims that they cause violence. If you are considering a trial of one of these drugs, you should know that there are no scientific data in children to verify these claims. In our clinic, we have used these agents in large numbers of children and found them highly effective with minimal concerns of behavioral activation and no cases of a sudden onset of severe

TABLE 15. The Preparation and Strengths of the Antidepressants

Medication		
Generic name	Brand name	Sizes and preparation

Selective serotonin reuptake inhibitors

Fluoxetine	Prozac	10, 20, 60 mg; capsules 20 mg/tsp; suspension
Sertraline	Zoloft	50, 100 mg; tablets 20 mg/cc; suspension
Fluvoxamine	Luvox	50, 100 mg; tablets
Paroxetine	Paxil	10, 20, 30, 40 mg; tablets 20 mg/5 cc suspension
Citalopram	Celexa	20, 40, mg; tablets
Escitalopram	Lexapro	10, 20 mg; tablets

Tricyclics

Desipramine	Norpramin Pertofrane	10, 25, 50, 75, 100, 150 mg; tablets
Nortriptyline	Pamelor Vivactyl	10, 25, 50 mg; capsules 10 mg/tsp; oral suspension
Imipramine	Tofranil	10, 25, 50, 75, 100, 150 mg; tablets and capsules
Amitriptyline	Elavil	10, 25, 50, 75, 100, 150 mg; tablets
Protriptyline	Vivactyl	5, 10 mg; tablets
Maprotiline	Ludiomil	25, 50, 75 mg; tablets
Clomipramine	Anafranil	25, 50, 100 mg; tablets

Atypical

Venlafaxine	Effexor	25, 37.5, 50, 75 mg; tablets 37.5, 75, 150 mg; extended-release tablets
Trazodone	Desyrel	50, 100, 150, 300 mg; tablets
Nefazodone	Serzone	100, 150, 200, 250 mg; tablets
Bupropion	Wellbutrin	75, 100 mg; tablets 100, 150, 200 mg; sustained-release tablets 150, 300 mg; extended-release tablets
Mirtazapine	Remeron	15, 30 mg; tablets
Doxepin	Sinequan	10, 25, 50, 75, 100, 150 mg; capsules 10 mg/cc; solution

(cont.)

TABLE 15. *(cont.)*

| Medication | | Sizes and preparation |
Generic name	Brand name	
Monamine oxidase inhibitors		
Phenelzine	Nardil	15 mg; tablets
Tranylcypromine	Parnate	10 mg; tablets

violence. Moreover, these medications have been studied extensively with an excellent track record.

If you read an August 3, 2003, *New York Times* article titled "Debate Resumes on the Safety of Depression's Wonder Drugs," you may also hesitate to approve treatment of your child with Paxil—and may again question the safety of the entire SSRI class of drugs. The article reported that unpublished studies had found that Paxil may actually cause children and teenagers to have thoughts of suicide. In controlled clinical trials of Paxil for depression carried out overseas, there was a higher risk for thinking about suicide (3%) compared to kids receiving a sugar pill (1.5%). Of note, there was no injury or death that resulted from treatment. However, in October 2003 the FDA sent out a health advisory warning doctors to exercise caution in prescribing the SSRIs for children and adolescents and to closely monitor those who do take these medications. In December of that year the Times reported that the British equivalent of the FDA had issued an even stronger warning, and in the U.S. public hearings are scheduled to follow up on such concerns in February 2004. All experts agree that, for a variety of reasons, it is extremely difficult to establish a link between the SSRIs and suicidal ideation or suicide attempts in young people.

There are lingering concerns in adults that antidepressants may transiently increase suicide thoughts, and this may be the case with Paxil for depression. In light of an absence of data indicating that Paxil is effective for depression, most doctors are not prescribing Paxil for depression in kids. Other related SSRIs such as Zoloft and Prozac have *not* been found to have a similar specific theoretical risk for suicide thoughts after initiation in clinical practice and have been reported to be effective for depression. It is also important to note that in the general population of adolescents almost one-quarter have suicidal thoughts, and that there has been a drastic decrease in suicidal behavior (attempts and completed suicides) thought, in part, to be related to the appropriate use of this class of medication. Our group recently reported that SSRIs can lead to behavioral side effects including more depression, etc., in 20% of cases; hence, you should observe your child carefully throughout the initiation of a new medication for *any* untoward side effects (including psychological).

Based on large, multiple-site studies of these agents in kids, the SSRIs are considered the first line of pharmacological treatment for depression, obsessive–compulsive disorder, selective mutism (not speaking in certain settings), and certain other anxiety disorders. Because of their effects on the body, these medications have fewer sedative, cardiovascular (blood pressure and EKG changes), and weight-gain side effects than other antidepressants. Although similar in their effects of making more serotonin available in regions of the brain, the SSRIs vary from one another in their chemical structures, breakdown rates in the body, and side effects. Often, when one SSRI proves ineffective for a child, another may be very effective.

The suggested daily doses of SSRIs for children have been similar to those for adults, but this is changing. A study that our group recently did with the makers of Prozac showed that 10 mg per day, versus the adult dose of 20 mg per day, was sufficient. For instance, children ages 6–12 who require Prozac for depression, anxiety, or obsessive–compulsive disorder should have this medication started at no more than 10 mg daily and slowly increased as necessary. While data are not available for other SSRI, given these data, it seems prudent to start younger children on one-half the dose of an adult starting dose.

Prozac lasts a long time in the body, approximately 7–9 days, whereas Zoloft and Luvox last about 24 hours. That is why it takes 1 month to reach a consistent blood level of Prozac and up to 2 months after discontinuing Prozac for it to leave the blood entirely. For the same reason, the shorter-acting SSRIs are the better choice for children who have the potential to become agitated or to swing toward mania because of the antidepressant effects. Children who are more likely to switch from depression to bipolar disorder include those with a family member with bipolar disorder, those with sudden onset of their depression, those with psychosis (hallucinations), and those who are already agitated. Should the medication need to be stopped, the shorter-acting medications will leave the bloodstream quickly and thus cut off any disabling effect.

The dosage range depends on which medication is prescribed for your child. In general, though, doses of the SSRIs are lower for depression and anxiety and relatively higher for obsessive–compulsive disorder.

Younger children (under 12 years) should be started at relatively lower doses of these medications than adolescents. For example, prepubertal children should be started at 10 mg of Prozac; in contrast, adolescents can start at 20 mg per day, like adults. Although more or less equally effective, Zoloft and Luvox require higher dosing than Celexa and Prozac because the former two are less potent (see page 224). Here are some guidelines:

- Prozac is typically dosed from 5 to 40 mg daily and is available in both capsule form (10 and 20 mg) and a liquid preparation (20 mg per 5 cc, which is equivalent to 1 teaspoon).
- The range of Zoloft dosing is from 50 to 200 mg daily. Zoloft comes in 50-mg and 100-mg tablets, which are scored and easily broken in half, and 20 mg per cc suspension.
- Luvox is dosed from 50 to 300 mg daily and also is available in scored 50-mg and 100-mg tablets.
- Celexa is dosed generally from 10 to 40 mg daily and is available in 20- and 40-mg tablets.
- Lexapro is generally dosed from 5 to 10 mg and comes in 10-mg tablets that can be broken.

All of the SSRIs can be given once daily, although parents sometimes note that their children respond better and tolerate the medications more fully when the shorter-acting compounds Zoloft and Luvox are prescribed in split doses twice a day. The SSRIs are generally administered in the morning, with the exception of Luvox, which may cause sedation and, if so, is better tolerated when given at night. Luvox is an excellent choice for depressed, obsessive, or anxious children who have marked sleep problems and can benefit from the sedative properties of the drug, usually noted 1–8 hours after administration.

The most common side effects of these medications include agitation, stomachaches and diarrhea (gastrointestinal symptoms), irritability, activation, headaches, and sleep disorders. We recently reported that emotional and behavioral side effects (e.g., activation, panic reaction, worse depression) emerged in 20% of kids taking the SSRIs. On average, these emotional or behavioral side effects started 3 months into treatment and typically abated with discontinuation of the SSRI. We also found that almost half of those kids who had a reaction to one SSRI (e.g., Prozac) had another reaction to another SSRI (e.g., Zoloft).

Some SSRIs alter the liver's ability to break down other medications, so *be sure to ask your child's doctor about the safety of taking any other medi-*

cations, including over-the-counter preparations. For example, Prozac is well known to increase blood levels of other medications such as tricyclic antidepressants and some medications used to control seizures. The FDA also cautions against the use of common antihistamines such as Tavist and certain antibiotics (like erythromycin) with some of these medications because of a theoretical drug interaction. To date, for children with seasonal allergies (hayfever), Claritin, Allegra, or Zyrtec appears to have the least such interaction.

Your child does not need to have cardiac monitoring or blood tests before or during treatment with the SSRIs. The drugs have no cardiovascular side effects, and blood levels of these medicines, vital signs, or routine blood monitoring are not used in clinical practice.

THE TRICYCLIC ANTIDEPRESSANTS

The tricyclic antidepressants include amitriptyline (Elavil), imipramine (Tofranil), desipramine (Norpramin), nortriptyline (Pamelor), doxepin, clomipramine (Anafranil), and protriptyline (Vivactyl). These medications are used primarily for ADHD and tic disorders and less frequently for anxiety and depression. They all act on children (and adults) in similar ways. Called *tricyclics* because of their chemical structure (three rings), they appear to work by making more of the neurotransmitters available for nerve-to-nerve communication. As with most classes of drugs, however, each medication has its unique aspects. For example, the effects of the antidepressants on certain neurotransmitters in the brain—in particular serotonin, norepinephrine, and dopamine—vary. In turn, the individual drugs vary in how well they improve various psychiatric problems. Different antidepressants also have different side effect profiles. Desipramine, for instance, because it causes less blockade of a body and brain chemical called *histamine* (antihistamine), causes less sedation and dry mouth in children than other medicines in this class, such as imipramine.

As with many other medications, children will vary widely in how they break down (metabolize) any tricyclic antidepressant they are taking. Therefore, there is no standard dosage for all children. Don't be surprised, though, if your child's dose ends up being the same one that you or another adult you know takes. As explained on page 100, children and adolescents have a more efficient metabolism than adults and may need more medication for their body weight than adults do. To determine how much of the medication is in your child's bloodstream and to avoid poten-

Why don't the tricyclic antidepressants work for depression in children?

We are not at all sure why the older generation of tricyclic antidepressants is not effective for depression in children and adolescents. Some notable observations suggest that in the studies testing these compounds many of the children receiving inactive placebos responded to treatment that erased the generally (but marginally) positive effect of the active tricyclic antidepressant. Some researchers have suggested that depression in youth may be very different at the neurotransmitter level from what is seen in adults. Since we think the medications work by altering neurotransmitter levels, some medicines, such as tricyclic antidepressants, may work better in adults than in children; others, such as the SSRIs (Prozac-like drugs), may work equally well; and others may prove to work better in children. Unfortunately, we have yet to discover that last group.

tial toxicity from a blood level that is too high, your child's doctor will check blood levels.

To start, the doctor will probably prescribe a 10-mg or 25-mg dose and increase it slowly every 4–5 days by 10–25 mg. Current practice, which varies from doctor to doctor, suggests that when an effective dose is reached, blood levels and an EKG should be obtained. Typical dose ranges for the tricyclic antidepressants are from 25 to 150 mg daily.

The tricyclic antidepressants are one option for children who suffer from insomnia or tics when their ADHD is treated with stimulants—11-year-old Gail found 25 mg of nortriptyline twice a day very effective in controlling her ADHD and allowing her to sleep better than she did on Metadate CD or Dexedrine—but these drugs also have side effects of their own. Common short-term adverse effects of the tricyclic antidepressants include dry mouth, constipation, sedation, headaches, vivid dreams, stomachaches, rash, and blurred vision. Gail reported dry mouth and occasional nightmares. Since the tricyclic antidepressants reduce the production of saliva and lead to a dry mouth, they may also promote tooth decay.

Children on these medications also may get a red, itchy rash, usually over the chest. Since the rash is not life-threatening, it is often possible to continue the medication as tolerated, with careful monitoring of the progress of the rash. Often 12.5–25 mg of Benadryl or Atarax will help reduce

> **What can I do for the dry mouth that bothers my daughter so much?**
>
> I suggest keeping a water bottle by your child's bed and allowing her to take sips of water throughout the day. Encourage your children to avoid candy with sugar since it will increase the potential for cavities.

the redness and itchiness. If the rash persists or worsens, the tricyclic antidepressant should be stopped.

Long-term use of the tricyclic antidepressants has no known negative effects. Headaches, stomach cramping, diarrhea, and vomiting may result from stopping the drugs suddenly, however, so tapering is recommended.

There are lingering concerns about cardiac risks associated with tricyclic antidepressants in children. The issue arose following several case reports of sudden death in children who were being treated with desipramine. One evaluation of this issue concluded that children who are taking desipramine may have a slightly increased risk of sudden death, but not much higher than that of children who are not taking medication. Parents should know, however, that the data evaluated were imprecise and the reports were plagued by uncertainty. The sad fact is that a number of unfortunate children die each year for unclear reasons, and the link suggested in these cases may simply have been a coincidence resulting from the fact that at that time many children were being treated with desipramine. This is not to say the tricyclic antidepressants have no effect on the heart. In fact, minor effects on the EKG are seen often, most commonly a speeding up of the heart (*tachycardia*) and slowing of the electrical impulses through the heart (*conduction delays*). Although this varies from practice to practice, many doctors have an EKG completed prior to starting a tricyclic antidepressant and order follow-up EKGs occasionally throughout treatment. If your child has a preexisting cardiac problem outside of a common heart murmur, you may want to ask your pediatrician about a consultation with a pediatric cardiologist before initiating treatment with a tricyclic antidepressant.

Far and away the greatest risk brought by tricyclic antidepressants is overdose. Because of the lethality of tricyclic antidepressant overdose, you must carefully store the medication so it is inaccessible to all the children in your family. Many parents rest easiest when the drug is locked away and the key is hidden. This goes for your own medications as well if you are taking antidepressants. Children have been known to take their parents' antidepressants, by mistake or intentionally to hurt themselves, so take every precaution to protect your family.

OTHER ANTIDEPRESSANTS

Several other antidepressants effective in adults are used frequently in children and adolescents. These medications are atypical in that their chemical structures and mechanism of action are different from the other antidepressants.

Wellbutrin (Bupropion)

Wellbutrin (bupropion) is a unique antidepressant. The Wellbutrin molecule looks similar to the stimulant preparation amphetamine, and the compound also resembles it in its effect on dopamine neurotransmission in the brain. This drug is helpful for ADHD and depression and is particularly useful in depressed children who have bad mood swings or in those in whom there are concerns about mania or behavioral activation with a medication. Buproprion may also be very helpful for ADHD or mood problems in adolescents with substance use problems. This medicine is also FDA-approved to help with smoking cessation in adults (called Zyban).

Wellbutrin works rapidly, peaking in the blood after 2 hours and lasting 8–14 hours. The usual dose range in children is from 37.5 to 300 mg per day in two or three divided doses. The sustained-release preparation (100, 150, and 200 mg) can be given once or twice daily. A new extended-release form (150 mg and 300 mg) can be given once in the morning.

Bupropion is relatively free of drug interactions with prescribed or over-the-counter medications. Bupropion is commonly used with a stimulant, for example. The major side effects in children include irritability, decreased appetite, insomnia, and worsening of tics. Irritability is often a flag that the dose needs to be reduced. Short-acting Wellbutrin also has a somewhat higher rate of drug-induced seizures (4 in 1,000 individuals) relative to other antidepressants, particularly in higher doses or in patients with untreated preexisting seizures or with bingeing and purging problems (bulimia). No EKG or laboratory monitoring is necessary during Wellbutrin therapy.

Effexor (Venlafaxine)

Effexor (venlafaxine) is similar to the SSRIs in its effect on enhancing serotonin in certain areas of the brain by blocking its reuptake, but also possesses some *noradrenergic* properties. It is thus known as an *SNRI (serotonin–norepinephrine reuptake inhibitor)*. While clinical use suggests that Effexor is helpful for depression in kids, like Paxil, it has not been systematically shown in clinical trials to beat placebos. Moreover, more infrequent cases of fleeting suicidality were seen in the Effexor group compared to placebos. Therefore, as with any medication, careful observation of your child while initiating and during the earlier phases of treatment for side effects is paramount.

Effexor is dosed from 12.5 mg up to a total of 225 mg daily in twice-a-day split dosing. An extended-release (XR) tablet is available, allowing once-a-day dosing. The medication's potential side effects are nausea during the initial stages of treatment, agitation, stomachaches, headaches, and, at higher doses, blood pressure elevation. No specific blood monitoring is required, but you should discuss the potential drug interactions with the doctor before your child starts on this drug.

> **noradrenergic:** Pertaining to the adrenergic nerves in the body. Noradrenaline is involved in many of the "automatic" activities in the body, such as heart rate control, as well as being involved in anxiety, mood, and inhibition control. Synonymous with *norepinephrine*.
>
> **split dose:** A dose meant for a single administration that is divided up for a two- or three-times-a-day regimen. Synonymous with *divided dose*.

Serzone (Nefazodone) and Desyrel (Trazodone)

These two drugs are related compounds and in recent years have been used to treat depression, anxiety, sleep problems, and nonspecific oppositionality in young people. Both Serzone and trazodone are relatively short-acting compounds lasting about 12 hours. In children and adolescents, trazodone is dosed from 25 to 200 mg and is generally given at night. Serzone dosing is less well established, with 25 to 400 mg daily typically being prescribed in split doses. Serzone may be helpful in kids with bipolar or bipolar-like problems with depression.Because of the sedative properties of trazodone, it has been used very successfully as a sleep agent at doses of 25–50 mg nightly. Common side effects of these medications include sedation, agitation, dry mouth, constipation, and confusion at higher doses. Serzone may rarely cause hepatitis (inflammation of the liver). In males, trazodone has been relegated to a second- or third-line drug of choice because it has been reported infrequently to cause the potentially serious difficulty of painful, sustained erections (priapism). No EKG or blood monitoring is necessary for either of these compounds.

Remeron (Mirtazapine)

Remeron is a unique antidepressant with serotonergic activity, used for depression in adults. Because of its sleep-promoting effects, Remeron is commonly prescribed for youth with depression and/or difficulty going to sleep (see page 262). The dosage is generally 7.5–15 mg nightly. Side effects include excess sedation, heaviness, and upset stomach.

Monoamine Oxidase Inhibitors

Another class of less commonly used antidepressants is called the *monoamine oxidase inhibitors* (MAOIs). MAOIs work by stopping the breakdown of norepinephrine and dopamine in the sending nerve (presynaptic neuron), making more of these compounds available for neurotransmission. While these drugs are among the oldest and most effective antidepressants, they impose strict dietary restrictions, which has severely limited their usefulness. Parnate (tranylcypromine) and Nardil (phenelzine) can be helpful in treating juvenile depression, anxiety, panic, and ADHD. Daily doses should be increased carefully based on response and adverse effects and range from 10 to 50 mg daily. Besides dietary restrictions, the major limitations on using these medications are drug interactions. Children and adolescents taking the drugs must avoid foods containing the amino acid tyramine (aged foods and most cheeses), certain drugs of abuse (cocaine and ecstasy), and most cold medicines, all of which can induce dangerous high blood pressure. *Be sure to go over the details of these adverse effects with your child's doctor before initiating this medication. While on these medications, children should avoid most other medications.* Short-term adverse effects in children include blood pressure swings with changes in position Oying to standing), weight gain, drowsiness, and dizziness. No EKG or blood monitoring is necessary.

Antidepressants in Development

As of early 2004, several new antidepressants were being developed. One that may or may not be on the market by the time this revised edition is in print is duloxetine (a medication made by Eli Lilly & Company, with no trade name designated yet). Duloxetine shares some similarities with venlfaxine (Effexor) in that it has both serotonergic and noradrenergic reuptake blockade effects. In testing being completed for the FDA in adults (no child studies), it appears to be a well tolerated and efficacious antidepressant. Again, no data are available in children, but presumably it will be tried on youth with depression, anxiety, and/or ADHD. Watch the Internet and other sources of reliable science reports for updates.

CHAPTER 14

THE MOOD STABILIZERS

The name of this class of medications describes what these drugs do for children: control the volatile emotional and behavioral swings that plague those with mood disorders. Not surprisingly, this group of drugs is the first-line pharmacology of choice for children with bipolar disorder or manic depression. The mood stabilizers also are used often in children who suffer from significant mood swings, overactivity, and aggressiveness. The most common of the mood stablizers is lithium, followed by various anticonvulsants.

LITHIUM CARBONATE

Lithium carbonate (Cibalith, Eskalith, Lithobid, Lithonate, Lithotabs) is one of the mainstays of treatment for juvenile bipolar disorders. Lithium is a salt, and it bears chemical similarities to sodium, potassium, calcium, and magnesium, which occur naturally in the human body. In fact, before its toxicity at high doses became apparent, lithium was used as a salt replacement for adults with high blood pressure. (Imagine the mellowing after-dinner effects on adults who salted their steak with lithium!) Although we don't know exactly how lithium works (as is the case with most psychotropic agents), it appears to operate at a cellular level, altering hormones and neurons.

In children and adolescents, lithium lasts about 18 hours in the bloodstream. However, with routine daily dosing, it will accumulate to some degree in the blood. Unlike the majority of psychotropic agents, lithium is broken down (metabolized) and cleared (excreted) exclusively in the kid-

TABLE 16. The Preparation and Strengths of the Mood Stabilizers

Medication		
Generic name	Brand name	Sizes and preparation
Lithium salts	Lithobid, Lithonate, Lithotabs, Eskalith, Cibalith	150, 300, 450 mg; tablets 8 mEq/tsp; suspension (= 300-mg tablet)
Carbamazepine	Tegretol, Carbachol	100, 200 mg; tablets 100 mg/tsp; suspension
Oxcarbazepine	Trileptal	150, 300, 600 mg; tablets
Valproic acid	Valproate, Depakote, Depakote ER, Depakene sprinkles	125, 250, 500 mg; tablets and capsules 250 mg/tsp; suspension
Gabapentin	Neurontin	100, 300, 400 mg; capsules 400, 600, 800 mg; tablets
Lamotrigine	Lamictal	25, 100, 150, 200 mg; tablets
Topiramate	Topamax	25, 100, 200 mg; tablets
Tiagabine	Gabitril	4, 12, 16, 20 mg; tablets

neys. Children and adults break the drug down in a similar fashion, though children's excretion of lithium is faster and more efficient.

It's important to monitor the amount of lithium in the child's blood to help in dosing for effectiveness and to avoid side effects and toxicity. As with other medications, your child will have to be on the same daily dose for about 5 days before reaching a "steady-state level" that will give an accurate reading of how much lithium is in the bloodstream. Samples for blood lithium determination should be drawn from the child approximately 12 hours after the last dose of lithium. Generally, lithium levels are drawn in the morning, with no lithium given to the child until after the sample is taken. (If lithium were administered directly before a blood sample, the blood reading could be reported as falsely high.) Usually your child's blood will be drawn from a vein (venipuncture), but for children in whom this method is a problem, some medical facilities offer finger stick measurements and saliva lithium levels.

The usual lithium starting dose ranges from 150 to 300 mg in twice-a-day dosing. In some children, lower doses are sufficient for control of mood instability, but some children may require more than 1,800 mg per day (six tablets) for adequate control of their mood. There is no firm agreed-on therapeutic blood lithium level in pediatric psychiatry. Suggested guidelines include serum levels of 0.6–1.5 mEq per liter for children with marked current problems and levels of 0.4–0.8 mEq per liter for maintenance or prophylactic (protective) therapy. *Nevertheless, as with any other intervention, the lowest effective dose and/or serum level should be used.* For example, I treat a 7-year-old girl with bipolar disorder who is doing well on 150 mg twice daily with a serum level of only 0.4 mEq per liter. Slow- or controlled-release lithium preparations are available (Lithobid, Lithotabs).

Lithium has a number of side effects. The more common short-term side effects include gastrointestinal symptoms such as nausea, vomiting, and upset stomach; central nervous symptoms such as tremor, sleepiness, and, rarely, memory impairment; and kidney symptoms, including increased urination (polyuria), leading to increased drinking of fluids (polydipsia).

An important point is that lithium essentially "tricks" the kidneys and produces a mild state of dehydration, which is why you will see your child drinking water so frequently. You should allow your child unlimited fluid and make arrangements for the school to do the same. Lithium can accumulate quickly in your child's blood, sometimes to a toxic level, during dehydration states. Toxic levels of lithium can damage the kidneys. Problems with walking or talking, tiredness, and seeing "weird colors" (especially around lights) are all signs of toxicity. *If your child is vomiting, has sustained diarrhea, or is not taking in a reasonable amount of fluid, contact the child's doctor.* In my practice, I will often ask parents to reduce the

---

How can we be sure our daughter gets the medication she needs when she keeps hiding the tablet in her cheek?

This is, unfortunately, a common ploy of children who, for whatever reason, do not want to take their medication. For these children—and for those who have difficulty swallowing tablets—lithium is available in a liquid form, lithium citrate. The liquid dose is roughly 1 teaspoon (5 cc), which is equivalent to the typical 300-mg tablet.

dose of lithium by half or not to give the lithium until the child is feeling better and taking in fluids appropriately.

Long-term use of lithium may alter your child's metabolism, causing substantial weight gain. Watch your child's diet and encourage exercise to control the weight gain. Other long-term side effects are decreased thyroid effectiveness, leading to hypothyroidism (low thyroid), and possible kidney damage. Information collected over the last 10 years, however, suggests that maintenance lithium therapy does not lead to serious kidney problems, at least in adults. Children should be checked by blood test to see how their thyroid and kidneys are working before lithium treatment is started, and these tests should be repeated approximately every 6 months while the child is on lithium.

Particular caution should be exercised if your child suffers from serious neurological, kidney, or heart disease. In addition, you should contact your child's practitioner if your child requires repeated nonsteroidal, antiinflammatory agents such as Advil or Motrin. Also, be sure to mention to any practitioner who may be starting another medication that your child is on lithium since there are a number of potential drug interactions. Often a repeat lithium level will be done if another medication with a potential drug interaction leading to increased blood lithium levels is added.

TEGRETOL/CARBACHOL

The anticonvulsants, also the treatment of choice for organic disorders such as temporal lobe epilepsy and brain injury, work as mood stabilizers by reducing abnormal firing of nerve impulses in the limbic regions (the emotional center) of the brain. The anticonvulsant medication Tegretol (carbamazepine) has been used to treat certain types of seizures in children for over 20 years and is often used in place of lithium or as a second-line drug of choice for mood instability.

Can I use the generic form of this anticonvulsant to save on cost?

The generic preparation, carbamazepine, has proven less well-formulated than the brand name Tegretol, being absorbed poorly and the tablets tending to fall apart, so I recommend the brand-name preparation and will use that name, Tegretol, throughout this section.

Tegretol is usually given in twice-a-day dosing and stays in the blood for about 16 hours. To reduce stomach irritation, it is commonly given with meals. The typical starting dose is 100 mg (in chewable form) to 200 mg daily up to a typical dose of 400–800 mg per day, depending on the amount in the blood and its effectiveness. The amount usually necessary in the blood to produce favorable effects without causing an excess of side effects is 4–12 mEq/L. Unfortunately, many children require higher doses and blood levels on the high side to maintain stability of their mood. Since the amount of medicine your child takes and the amount that is actually in the blood varies among individuals, close blood level monitoring is necessary. Tegretol is broken down extensively by the liver, and the amount in the blood may be either increased or decreased by other medications. Because of these complications and some potentially serious side effects, your child's blood should be monitored before starting on Tegretol, generally after 6 weeks, and then at least twice a year, for liver and blood counts as well as to check Tegretol levels.

The side effects that Tegretol may cause are unfortunately fairly broad in scope. The most common short-term side effects include drowsiness, nausea, vomiting, dizziness, and blurred or double vision, particularly at higher doses and blood levels. In addition, Tegretol may reduce the number of white blood cells and therefore your child's ability to fight infection. A simple blood test to determine the white blood cell count is advised any time your child develops a serious sore throat or other infection. Reactions such as liver toxicity and skin disorders, including a rash or a more serious type involving the inside of the mouth and the palms of the hands (Stevens–Johnson syndrome), have been reported but appear to be rare.

VALPROIC ACID

Valproic acid (brand names Valproate, Depakene, and, most common, Depakote) is often used as a first-line agent for the treatment of bipolar disorders in children and adolescents. Valproic acid is an anticonvulsant-class agent (treats seizures) and is FDA-approved for the treatment of bipolar disorder in adults. Depakote is broken down by the liver and lasts about 8–16 hours in the blood. A typical blood level is between 50 and 100 mEq/L, although some doctors will push blood levels to 130 mEq/L for children who have seizures that don't respond readily to treatment, severe mood instability, or behavioral outbursts. Children are generally started on 125–250 mg daily, and from there the dose is increased as necessary to achieve a "therapeutic" blood level. A new form of valproic acid, Depakote ER, is available that can be given once or twice a day in children and, like Depakote is very helpful for bipolar disorder. Since Depakote ER is slightly less potent, your child's doctor will need to increase the amount of Depakote ER relative to Depakote your child was receiving.

The ultimate dosage will vary greatly from child to child, depending on how each one breaks down the medication. Complicating the dosing further, Depakote will actually increase its *own* breakdown. Therefore, to arrive at a safe but effective blood level of the drug, many doctors request frequent blood levels during the initial phases of treatment. Your child will definitely need to have a blood test to determine blood counts and liver function before treatment begins and approximately every 6 months during treatment with the drug. Some children may require more than 1,500–2,000 mg a day to sustain a reasonably effective level of Depakote.

Common short-term side effects include sedation, nausea, dizziness, loss of appetite, and weight gain. Rarely, Depakote may cause a reduction in the blood count or may cause a mild and generally nondangerous inflammation of the liver (hepatitis), which is often picked up only on routine blood studies and resolves spontaneously. The risk of serious liver problems appears to be increased when Depakote is used with other antiseizure medications, particularly in children under age 10. Depakote may also rarely cause a painful swelling of the pancreas, although no specific monitoring is required.

Valproic acid has been reported to be associated with polycystic ovary syndrome, a condition characterized by painful ovarian cysts, increased testerosterone, and obesity. In fact, some doctors avoid its use in adolescent girls. Another look at that data, however, seems to indicate that being obese and having bipolar disorder are the biggest risk factors for this uncommon condition and that other medications share a similar risk for causing obesity—and possible polycystic ovaries. Despite many years of use, our group has not had any patient develop polycystic ovaries, and we continue to use Valproate regularly.

OTHER ANTICONVULSANTS USED FOR MOOD STABILIZATION: LAMICTAL, TRILEPTAL, TOPAMAX, NEURONTIN, GABITRIL

A new generation of anticonvulsant medications that are also mood-stabilizing medications has been used in children and adolescents with aggression, agitation, self-injurious behavior, and most commonly mood lability and bipolar disorder. While undergoing testing currently for their efficacy and tolerability in juvenile bipolar disorder, controlled data derived from studies of adults and smaller open studies in kids indicate that Lamictal (lamotriine), rileptal (oxcarbazepine), Topamax (topirimate), and Neurontin (gabapentin) may be important agents to add to the armamentarium of medications used for kids.

Lamictal is another mood stabilizer, also used for complex partial seizures, that in adults has been FDA-pproved for the treatment of depression in bipolar disorder. Lamictal is an extremely good medication for treating depression in youth with bipolar disorder *without* activating mania. Lamictal is often added to other medications for bipolar disorder such as Depakote. Like Depakote and Tegretol, Lamictal has a number of drug interactions, so your child's blood levels should be monitored. Major side effects of Lamictal are a skin rash, which can be serious, blurred and double vision, tiredness, and dizziness. In adults, typical dosing of Lamictal is 150–250 mg twice daily. At the time of this writing, dosing for childhood mood instability has not been established, although we typically use between 150 and 300 mg daily. The dose of Lamictal should be increased very slowly in weekly increments by no more than 25 mg to avoid the risk of a rash. The rash associated with Lamictal can be of two major types: (1) a more minor rash that is typically on the trunk of the child that occurs in up to one out of ten children, and (2) a very serious rash, necessitating emergency care, that affects not only the body but the mouth, hands, and feet of the child with blisters and loss of skin.

Sally is a 14-year-old girl with bipolar disorder. She noted feeling depressed but did not manifest mania on Risperdal 1 mg twice daily with Depakote ER 1,000 mg every morning. An increase in both the Risperdal and Depakote was not helpful. Lamictal was started at 25 mg and increased to 100 mg over 4 weeks. She noted a dramatic improvement in the depression as well as reduced overall irritability.

Trileptal is a sibling medication of Tegretol (carbamazepine) that has been very helpful for the management of aggression and the manic symptoms of bipolar disorder. Trileptal is dosed starting with 150–300 mg daily and increased in twice-a-day dosing to a typical dose of 1,200 mg per day in a younger child and up to a maximum of 2,400 mg per day in an adolescent. Like other anticonvulsants, it may take from 4 to 6 weeks to see the full therapeutic benefit of Trileptal unfold.

Trileptal has few drug interactions. Side effects mostly commonly include nausea, dizziness, and tiredness. Your child should have her blood checked for a sodium level, as this medication rarely can cause a reduced blood sodium level (hyponatremia).

Topamax (topiramate) is another anticonvulsant that has been predominately used for stabilization of weight in children who have drug-induced weight gain with the medications for bipolar disorder. Often, Topamax is added to a regimen of an antipsychotic or anticonvulsant at doses of 25–100 mg twice daily with good effects to keep weight off, as well as assist youth who have gained massive amounts of weight due to their medications. We have seen some children shed 60 pounds when being treated with Topamax in addition to their other medications. Moreover, some data in adults suggest that Topamax is a viable treatment for bulimia.

Side effects of Topamax include dulling of thinking processes at relatively higher doses (more than 100 mg per day) that can limit its use. Rarely Topamax can cause children to overheat—in part related to the lack of sweating. Parents should observe children on this medication during strenuous activities in the heat to ensure that they are adequately hydrated and do not appear overheated. Other side effects are more nuisance in nature and include sedation and dizziness. A blood test for your child's acid–base status should be completed infrequently.

Little is known about the anticonvulsant Kepra for behavioral disturbances; however, Neurontin used to be highly touted as an agent that is helpful for bipolar disorder but without substantial side effects. Unfortunately, no clinical trials have been completed in children, and five controlled trials in adults have failed to demonstrate efficacy compared to placebo for bipolar disorder. Despite these negative findings, largely because of its very benign side effect profile, clinicians continue to use Neurontin in less severe cases of bipolar disorder or more mild moodiness. Like lithium, Neurontin is broken down by the kidneys, so there is relatively little chance of drug interactions with the bulk of medications, which are metabolized by the liver. It appears to be extremely well tolerated and does not require intensive blood monitoring. Dosing of Neurontin usually starts at 300 mg twice daily up to 600–900 mg twice daily, with dizziness and sedation the most common side effects. Kepra has been evaluated in children with seizures and by nature of its mechanism of action appears to be an excellent candidate for study. Our preliminary use of the compound is very optimistic.

Also relatively new on the anticonvulsant scene and just being tried in children with bipolar disorder or marked moodiness is Gabitril. Like

Topamax, it is FDA-approved for adolescents for seizures but is being used in children as well. The maximum recommended daily dose of Gabitril is 32 mg. Since dosing information is based on adolescents with seizures, dosing of these medications should start low and be increased slowly until a positive effect to the medicine is noted or the maximum allowable dose is reached. Gabitril may cause dizziness, tiredness, and an unstable gait. Also like Topamax, Gabitril may interact with other drugs, so be sure to inform your child's primary-care doctor that your child is receiving these agents.

CHAPTER 15

THE ANXIETY-BREAKING MEDICATIONS

Like the mood stabilizers, the anxiety-reducing medications are categorized by the effect they have in children. Also called *anxiolytics,* they are used to treat the wide range of anxiety and panic disorders that share the predominant symptoms of worrying, nervousness, and anxiety. They are also used as adjunct treatment for tics and for sleep. Childhood anxiety disorders are relatively common and bear some similarities to the adult anxiety disorders.

> **anxiolytic:** A class of medications used to reduce ("lyse") anxiety.

Your child's practitioner will probably elect to try an SSRI (e.g., Luvox, Zoloft, Paxil) for your child's anxiety as a first-line agent. Because of their safety and effectiveness, benzodiazepines are also used for uncomplicated juvenile anxiety disorders. In some children who have severe anxiety conditions or a co-occurring disorder, combined treatment (such as an SSRI antidepressant or an atypical antipsychotic and a benzodiazepine) may be necessary.

THE BENZODIAZEPINES

The most common class of medications used to treat anxiety are the benzodiazepines. Among medications in this class of agents are Valium (diazepam), Librium (chlordiazepoxide), and Klonopin (clonazepam). The newer-generation, benzodiazepine-like medications include Xanax (alprazolam) and Buspar (buspirone).

The benzodiazepines and some of their breakdown products are active compounds; that is, these compounds directly affect the human body. Of interest, the liver breaks down most of the benzodiazepines into the

TABLE 17. The Preparation and Strengths of the Anxiety-Breaking Medications

Medication		
Generic name	Brand name	Sizes and preparation
Antihistamines		
Diphenhydramine	Benadryl	25, 50 mg; tablets 25 mg/tsp; suspension
Hydroxyzine	Vistaril, Atarax	25, 50 mg; tablets 2 mg/tsp; suspension
Chlorpheniramine maleate	Chlor-Trimeton	2, 4, 8 mg; tablets
Benzodiazepines (partial list)		
Clonazepam	Klonopin	0.5, 1, 2 mg; tablets
Alprazolam	Xanax	0.25, 0.5, 1 mg; tablets
Triazolam	Halcion	0.5, 1, 2 mg; tablets
Lorazepam	Ativan	0.5, 1 mg; tablets
Oxazepam	Serax	15, 30 mg; tablets
Diazepam	Valium	2, 5, 10 mg; tablets
Clorazepate	Tranxene	3.75, 7.5, 15 mg; capsules
Chlordiazepoxide	Librium	10, 25 mg; capsules
Atypical		
Buspirone	Buspar	5, 10, 15 mg; tablets

same compound in the blood, nordiazepam (note the similarity with the chemical name of Valium—diazepam).

THE PSYCHOTROPIC MEDICATIONS

The benzodiazepines act mainly on the central nervous system (brain), affecting a type of receptor called the *GABA receptor.* Barbiturates (*sedatives*) and alcohol have similar effects on this receptor, which is why all three are considered sedative in nature and can be used to stop withdrawal from one another. For instance, it is common practice to use Librium or Serax (oxazepam) to treat symptoms of withdrawal from alcohol.

> **sedative:** A sleep-producing agent.

In general, the benzodiazepines all have similar effects on anxiety, and the level of all of them peaks in the blood in 1–3 hours following a dose. Where they differ is in their sedative side effects and their strength. Panic and types of anxiety require a lot of antianxiety medication, so the stronger (more potent) benzodiazepines have been increasingly used in young people. In recent years, the strong (*high-potency*) benzodiazepines, Xanax and Klonopin, have received increasing attention as effective and safe treatments for anxiety and panic disorder with and without agorapho-

---

The pharmacist tells me my son's prescription is for a schedule IV controlled substance, and now I'm worried that he'll get addicted to his medication. Should I be concerned?

All sedatives, including benzodiazepines, can produce both physiological (body) and psychological dependence. However, addiction is generally a danger only when these substances are abused. Given that there is little abuse of these medications by children taking them legitimately, your child has a very small likelihood of becoming addicted to any of the benzodiazepines. If your child's doctor prescribes an anxiety-breaking medication over a period of more than 6 months, you need to balance the very small chance of addiction against the risk of not treating your child's anxiety disorder. Young people whose anxiety is not treated may try to medicate themselves by turning to alcohol and street drugs.

bia (difficulty leaving the house). Klonopin is a long-acting benzodiazepine given one to three times a day (usually twice a day) with a typical daily dose of 0.5–3 mg. Klonopin may take up to 2 hours to work. Xanax and Ativan, other high-potency benzodiazepines, work faster (within 30 minutes) but wear off more quickly and consequently are dosed more often during the day. The typical dose of Ativan and Xanax is 0.5–3 mg daily, similar to Klonopin. The intermediate-acting, midpotency benzodiazepines (Valium, Tranxene) work within 30 minutes and are also given three or four times a day because of the wearoff. Typical dosing is 2.5–20 mg daily.

In general, serious toxic effects of the benzodiazepines are virtually nonexistent (when used appropriately). The most commonly encountered short-term side effects are sedation, drowsiness, and decreased mental *acuity* (sharpness). Children may also have paradoxical response to the benzodiazepines. Instead of becoming less anxious or sedated (if used for sleep), they may get agitated and disinhibited. Disinhibited children may be silly, agitated, talkative, and overactive, become more anxious, sleep poorly (insomnia). Generally, if your child is the unlucky one to have this reaction, it will last for only a couple of hours. Rarely, benzodiazepines can cause or initiate a depression. With the exception of the small potential risk for dependence, the benzodiazepines have no known long-term, adverse effects. No baseline laboratory tests are necessary, and there is no need for blood monitoring with treatment.

> **disinhibition:** Loss of normal restraint or censorship of impulses and urges.

Long-term use of these medications may lead to tolerance, however. When the child's body gets used to the medication, more of it may become necessary to reduce the symptoms of anxiety. Stopping the medication abruptly, especially at higher doses, may lead to withdrawal. Withdrawal symptoms include agitation, edginess, sweating, and anxiety. More severe symptoms may include increased blood pressure, confusion, and seizures. The good news is that tapering off the drugs rather than stopping them abruptly can easily prevent withdrawal symptoms.

> **tolerance:** The loss of a response, either behavioral or physical, to a medication over a sustained period of time.

BUSPAR

Buspar (buspirone) is also an anxiety-breaking compound. Buspirone may be effective in the treatment of aggressive behaviors in children with developmental disorders, including pervasive developmental disorders. Buspar may also benefit kids with ADHD. Often Buspar is used in conjunction with the SSRIs (like Prozac) for anxiety or to boost the antidepressant's effect on depression.

Unlike the benzodiazepines, Buspar does not have anticonvulsant, sedative, or muscle-relaxant properties. Instead, the anxiety-breaking effect of Buspar may relate to reduction in serotonergic neurotransmission. Clinical experience with this drug suggests that it is not as effective as typical benzodiazepines; however, it also has significantly fewer side effects and a lower potential for abuse or dependence. Side effects include sedation, confusion, and disinhibition. Buspar is used at a dose range of 5–15 mg three times a day and does not require blood monitoring.

CHAPTER 16

THE ANTIHYPERTENSIVES

The antihypertensives—clonidine, guanfacine, and propranolol—are so named because they are used to treat high blood pressure in adults. In children and adolescents, they are used psychiatrically to treat tic disorders, ADHD, severe developmental disorders such as autism, and sleep problems. These medications may also reduce behaviors that place children at risk for harming themselves or others, such as severe outbursts or aggressivity. The antihypertensives are commonly used in combination with other agents such as the stimulants, mood stabilizers, and antidepressants.

CLONIDINE

Clonidine (Catapres) has become increasingly prominent in the psychopharmacological treatment of children, in part because of its wide range of usefulness and relative safety. In addition to ADHD and sleep disturbances, clonidine is now considered a first-line treatment in Tourette's disorder and other tic disorders. In addition, reports indicate that clonidine helps control aggression in children and adolescents with autism, pervasive developmental disorder, and other less well-described developmental disorders. Two recent studies have shown the added utility of clonidine with methylphenidate (stimulants) for the treatment of youth with tic disorders or Tourette's disorder and ADHD. Clonidine works in the brain by dampening one of the major chemical transmitter systems in the brain, the adrenergic nervous system. More specifically, it affects the release of norepinephrine, and hence nerve-to-nerve communication, in certain areas of the brain.

TABLE 18. The Preparation and Strengths of the Antihypertensives

Medication		
Generic name	Brand name	Sizes and preparation
Clonidine	Catapres	0.1, 0.2, 0.3 mg; tablets 1, 2, 3; skin patch
Guanfacine	Tenex	1 mg; tablet
Propranolol	Inderal	10, 20, 40, 60, 80 mg; tablets 20, 60, 120 mg; sustained-release tablets
Nadolol	Corgard	20, 40, 80, 120, 160 mg; tablets

> **adrenergic nervous system** : The complex set of
> nerves that use norepinephrine-based messengers and
> connect extensively with multiple organs in the body,
> including the heart, lungs, and hormone-producing glands.

Clonidine is a relatively short-acting compound, working for about 4 hours in children, so some kids need to take it up to four times a day. The amount necessary for effective treatment of tics and ADHD varies substantially among children, however. Clonidine comes as 0.1-, 0.2-, and 0.3-mg tablets, and therapy is usually started at the lowest possible dose of a half or quarter tablet of 0.1 mg, depending on the size of the child, and increased depending on the child's positive response and any adverse effects. At first it's best to give clonidine in the evening or before bed since it often causes sedation. In fact, the drug can be very helpful to children with sleep disturbances commonly associated with ADHD or the stimulants used to treat it. For sleep, children usually require at least half of a 0.1-mg tablet about 30 minutes before bedtime. A study from our group showed that clonidine was extremely helpful for over 80% of children with sleep problems after 3 years of follow-up, but apparently children develop some tolerance to its sedating properties since the average dose after 3 years was 0.15 mg (1½ 0.1-mg tablets).

One drawback of having to take clonidine several times a day is that your child may suffer ups and downs. An alternative designed to solve this problem is a skin patch (*transdermal* preparation), available in all three strengths, that can be worn around the clock. Unfortunately, skin irritation at the site of the patch is common, limiting this form of delivery.

> My son has a much smoother day with the clonidine skin patch,
> but what can I do about the nasty rash he's developed where
> the patch goes?
>
> These skin patches very commonly cause an inflammation (*dermatitis*)
> wherever they are placed on the skin. Two ways to avoid this troubling
> side effect are to move the patch to another spot on the body every day
> or to apply 0.5% hydrocortisone ointment, which can be purchased over
> the counter, to the skin area before putting the patch on your child.

---

transdermal : Absorbed through the skin.

The sedation that can be so helpful with sleep problems is the most common short-term side effect of clonidine. If your child is severely sedated, reducing the dose to a quarter of a tablet may be necessary, but be aware that sedation usually subsides with continued treatment. Clonidine can also produce irritability and depression. At doses of 0.4 mg daily and up, it may cause confusion. Recently, there was a report that three children receiving combinations of clonidine and other medications died for unclear reasons. However, further information indicated that there were many other extenuating circumstances surrounding the deaths, leading many experts to the conclusion that clonidine was not the main culprit. Clonidine itself is not known to be associated with long-term serious adverse effects. Surprisingly, despite being a powerful blood pressure medication in adults, clonidine has little effect on children's blood pressure. *However, abrupt withdrawal of clonidine has been associated with rebound high blood pressure, so slow tapering is advised.* In addition, caution should be exercised when clonidine is used with propranolol or other beta blocker agents—as it might be to treat severe behavioral outbursts, to treat children who are having marked sleep problems along with outbursts, or for children with blood pressure problems who need to be treated for hyperactivity/impulsivity and aggression associated with ADHD and/or comorbid conduct problems—because an adverse interaction has been reported.

Clonidine may be combined with stimulants for kids with severe ADHD and aggression, kids with tic disorders and ADHD, or for sleep problems in kids with ADHD. A recent large study indicated clonidine's effectiveness for ADHD and tics when combined with Ritalin.

> ### What are the differences between clonidine and Tenex?
>
> The two drugs have significant differences that will help determine which one is chosen for your child. In treating ADHD, Tenex appears to have a slightly better effect on attentional difficulties, while clonidine works better on hyperactivity or aggression. Clonidine is approximately 10 times more potent (stronger) than Tenex, but Tenex causes less sedation and irritability.
>
> Tenex comes in 1.0-mg tablets, and the typical starting dose is one-half tablet twice daily. Although established dosing parameters are not yet available for Tenex, it has been used up to 1.0 mg four times a day safely and effectively. The major side effects include irritability, tiredness, confusion at higher doses, and, rarely, agitation. Like clonidine, Tenex should not be discontinued abruptly, due to the risk of a transient rebound upward swing in your child's blood pressure.

TENEX

Another adult blood pressure medication that has little effect on children's blood pressure when given daily, Tenex (guanfacine) recently has emerged as a potentially useful agent for ADHD, tic and Tourette's disorders, and, to a lesser extent, nonspecific aggression. Although Tenex has not been studied as well as clonidine, it appears to operate in the same areas of the brain, affecting similar nerve-to-nerve communication. As with clonidine, studies have shown its usefulness and tolerability when combined with Ritalin for the treatment of kids with ADHD plus tic disorders.

PROPRANOLOL AND OTHER BETA BLOCKERS

The beta blockers are commonly used in medicine to control blood pressure and, to a lesser extent, behavior. Although not systematically investigated in children, beta blockers have been reported to be helpful in individuals with brain injury and severe impulse and control problems. Propranolol has also received considerable attention for its usefulness in the overactivity (*akathisia*) sometimes induced by the stimulants or antipsychotics, in phobias such as fear of speaking in front of others, and in self-abusive behaviors.

Propranolol is one of the most frequently prescribed and oldest beta blockers. Other medications of the beta blocker type that are similar to propranolol include atenolol, pindolol, and nadolol. Propranolol works by blocking areas of the adrenergic nervous system, specifically the set of receptors called the *beta-adrenergic receptors,* at multiple sites in the body. This in turn dampens the nerve-to-nerve communication. Propranolol also crosses the blood–brain barrier, and this probably accounts for some of its usefulness in reducing certain behaviors.

Propranolol is relatively short-lived, working for only about 4–6 hours after being taken. Dosages vary among children but usually start at 10 mg daily and increase as necessary every week to 2 weeks up to a maximum of approximately 200–300 mg per day with careful attention to side effects at higher doses.

Short-term adverse effects of propranolol are usually not serious and generally disappear when the medication is stopped. Nausea, vomiting, constipation, and mild diarrhea have been reported. Children also report vivid dreams, depression, and, rarely, hallucinations. Propranolol can cause slowing of the heart and reduced blood pressure, particularly at higher doses, so your child will need to have periodic blood pressure and pulse (vital sign) checks, which can be done at home. Be sure your child's doctor knows about any cardiac problems the child has, because propranolol should be avoided in certain cardiac conditions. Propranolol may also cause worsening of types of breathing problems (high airway resistance, wheezing) and thus should not be used in children who have asthma. Propanolol should also be used cautiously in children with diabetes since it may mask any underlying emergency warning signs of dangerously low blood sugars. No long-term effects of continued use of propranolol are known, but gradual tapering is recommended to prevent a rebound swing in your child's blood pressure.

CHAPTER 17

THE ANTIPSYCHOTICS

The antipsychotics are the only drugs available that treat psychosis effectively, but they are also more commonly used to treat other disorders in children such as substantial mood lability when more standard treatments have failed. Also called *major tranquilizers* or *neuroleptics,* these drugs have a history of substantial side effects. That is why they are generally reserved for more severely disturbed children and those who don't respond to other medications. Therefore, it is wise for you and your child's doctor to choose them only with a clear understanding of what they are being used for and the proposed length of time your child will be receiving them.

These medications are generally reserved as second-line drugs of choice for the treatment of Tourette's disorder, marked mood swings or moodiness (mood lability), as well as severely disruptive, self-injurious, or aggressive behaviors. They are the drug of choice for psychoses such as schizophrenia and the impairments in reality sometimes seen with depression or bipolar disorder (manic–depression) in kids. Increasingly, the newer-generation antipsychotics are being used earlier in the treatment of juveniles with severe and out-of-control moodiness (mania).

One problem you should be aware of when an antipsychotic is chosen as a second or third choice for one disorder is that it may still fail to address a commonly co-occurring disorder. Haldol (haloperidol) and Orap (pimozide), for example, are prescribed when Strattera, clonidine, and the tricyclic antidepressants fail to improve Tourette's disorder. While they may be very useful in reducing tics, they could have only limited effects on the obsessive–compulsive disorders and ADHD that often accompany Tourette's disorder.

Another cautionary note on how and when to choose antipsychotics: These drugs have also traditionally been used to control symptoms of agitation, aggression, and self-injurious behaviors in children with developmental disorders including mental retardation and pervasive developmental disorders (autism and autism-like disorders). Tradition, however, should not always rule. Here it is prudent to try medications with fewer side effects, including propranolol and clonidine, first. If you and the doctor do conclude that an antipsychotic should be tried, know the differences among them: while a more sedating, lower-potency agent such as Thorazine, Mellaril, or Seroquel may be beneficial for the more agitated child or adolescent, a more potent agent such as Trilafon, Navane, or Risperdal may be helpful for children who are having active hallucinations.

The antipsychotics are more or less similar in their pharmacological profiles and in their ability to treat psychosis, behavioral control, and other psychiatric disturbances (i.e., their efficacy). However, as shown in Table 19, they differ substantially in their strength (potency) and side effects (especially in causing muscular spasms and sedation). The major classes of traditional antipsychotic drugs used clinically are (1) the weaker, or low-potency, compounds (requiring higher dosages) such as Thorazine (chlorpromazine) and Mellaril (thioridazine); (2) the middle-strength compounds such as Stelazine (trifluoperazine), Navane (thiothixene), Trilafon (perphenazine), and Loxitane (loxapine); and (3) the strong, high-potency agents such as Haldol (haloperidol), Prolixin (perfenazine), and Orap (pimozide). There are also newer antipsychotic agents, including Clozaril (clozapine), Risperdal (risperidone), Zyprexa (olanzapine), Seroquel (quetiapine), Geodon (ziprasidone), and Abilify (aripiprazole). It is important to know as much as possible about the individual drugs before agreeing to any prescription of antipsychotics for your child.

The traditional antipsychotics such as Mellaril appear to work by blocking specific dopamine receptors (dopamine 2 type). Some of the side effects of these drugs result from their blocking other receptors as well: histamine, which results in the dry mouth and sedation characteristic of antihistamines; and the cholinergic system, which results in an increased heart rate and constipation. The newer atypical antipsychotic agents have less effect on other receptors and affect different dopamine receptors (see page 29).

TABLE 19. Preparation and Strengths of the Antipsychotics

Medication		
Generic name	Brand name	Sizes and preparation
Atypical (newest)		
Ziprasidone	Geodon	20, 40, 60, 80 mg; tablets
Aripiprazole	Abilify	5, 10, 15, 20, 30 mg; tablets
Risperidone	Risperdal	0.25, 0.5, 1, 2, 3 mg; tablets
Clozapine	Clozaril	25, 50, 100 mg; tablets
Olanzapine	Zyprexa	2.5, 5, 7.5, 10, 15 mg; tablets
Quetiapine	Seroquel	25, 100, 200 mg; tablets
High potency		
Haloperidol	Haldol	0.5, 1, 2, 5, 10, 20 mg; tablets 2 mg/ml; suspension
Pimozide	Orap	2 mg; tablet
Fluphenazine	Prolixin	1, 2.5, 5, 10 mg; tablets 5 mg/ml; suspension
Medium potency		
Trifluoperazine	Stelazine	1, 2, 5, 10 mg; tablets
Perphenazine	Trilafon	2, 4, 8, 16 mg; tablets
Thiothixene	Navane	1, 2, 5, 10, 20 mg; tablets 5 mg/ml; suspension
Loxapine	Loxitane	5, 10, 25, 50 mg; tablets 5 mg/tsp; suspension
Low potency		
Molindone	Moban	5, 10, 25, 50, 100 mg; tablets 4 mg/tsp; suspension
Mesoridazine	Serentil	10, 25, 50, 100 mg; tablets 25 mg/tsp; suspension
Thioridazine	Mellaril	10, 15, 25, 50, 100, 200 mg; tablets 5, 6, 20 mg/tsp; suspension
Chlorpromazine	Thorazine	10, 25, 50, 100, 200 mg; tablets 5, 6, 20 mg/tsp; suspension

DOSING

The usual dosage of antipsychotic drugs ranges between 25 and 300 mg daily for the low-potency agents such as Mellaril, Thorazine, Seroquel, or Clozaril; between 4 and 40 mg daily for the midpotency agents such as Trilafon, Stelazine, or Zyprexa; and between 0.5 and 6 mg daily for the high-potency agents such as Haldol, Prolixin, and Risperdal. Antipsychotic medications last a relatively long time in the blood and do not need to be given more than two times a day.

Most antipsychotic preparations are available in either tablet or capsule form. In addition, at least one compound from each class of antipsychotics is available in a liquid concentrate. Several compounds, including Thorazine, Haldol, Prolixin, and Geodon are available in injection form (injectable/intramuscular). Haldol and Prolixin are also available in an oily suspension (Decanoate), which is administered as an injection (intramuscular) that lasts from 2 weeks to 1 month. Orally dissolving tablets of Zyprexa and Risperdal are available and can be invaluable for children who may be hiding medication in their mouth but not swallowing it (cheeking) and who spit it out later. These preparations dissolve in the mouth and cannot be cheeked.

SIDE EFFECTS

Common short-term, reversible side effects of antipsychotic drugs are drowsiness, increased appetite, and weight gain. Certain side effects like dizziness, dry mouth, congested nose, and blurred vision are more commonly seen with the low-potency agents such as Thorazine. High-potency agents such as Haldol, Orap, and Abilify are more commonly associated with a set of side effects affecting various muscle groups (*extrapyramidal effects*) leading to muscle tightness and spasm (*dystonia*), rolling eyes, and restlessness leading to the inability to stay seated (*akathisia*). All antipsychotics may also cause a reversible Parkinson-like picture characterized by general slowing, tremor, tenseness, and a masked face.

Although visually bothersome to others, and sometimes uncomfortable for the child, many of the short-term side effects of the antipsychotics can be managed. Excessive sedation can be avoided by using less sedating antipsychotics (Risperdal, Geodon, or Abilify instead of Thorazine, Seroquel, or Zyprexa) and managed by prescribing most of the daily dose at night either with dinner or at bedtime. Drowsiness should not be confused with impaired thinking and can usually be corrected by adjusting the dose and timing of administration. In fact, antipsychotics cause little to no mental confusion or impairment when used in low doses. Certain side effects such as dry mouth, constipation, and blurred vision can be minimized by choosing a medium- or high-potency compound (Stelazine, Navane, Haldol, or Risperdal instead of Thorazine or Mellaril). Muscular spasms (extrapyramidal reactions) can be avoided in most cases by slowly increasing these medications or using a lower-potency, weaker agent such as Navane or Stelazine instead of Haldol or Orap.

In our clinic, we tend to avoid Haldol or Prolixin in children because of these muscle spasms, which, although bothersome, are not dangerous. If, however, your child *is* responding well to a particular antipsychotic and has the muscular spasms, a class of safe medications (anti-Parkinson agents) can be added just for the side effects. The agents useful for these spasms include over-the-counter Benadryl for the short term, if relief is needed immediately, or prescribed Cogentin or amantidine to be taken daily for the long haul. If your child is on antipsychotics and develops agitation with an inability to sit still, the possibility that this is a side effect of the medication should be considered. Similar to treating muscular spasms, Benadryl, Cogentin, amantadine, the beta blockers (such as propranolol), and the benzodiazepines (Klonopin) may be helpful in eliminating these side effects.

Another very infrequent but severe reaction to antipsychotic agents is *neuroleptic malignant syndrome.* This reaction consists of severe muscle tightness, confusion, sweating, fever, and instability of blood pressure and pulse. *If you see anything resembling these symptoms in your child, contact your physician immediately or take your child to the emergency room.* If neuroleptic malignant syndrome is suspected, blood tests should be completed to help determine if there has been any muscle or kidney damage. Treatment of neuroleptic malignant syndrome requires intensive medical surveillance and consists of immediate stopping of the drug.

As in adults, the long-term use of antipsychotic drugs in children and adolescents may be associated with a feared, often irreversible, side effect called *tardive dyskinesia.* Tardive dyskinesia is a group of movements that the child is not able to stop entirely. It often starts as lip smacking and tongue rolling and may progress to involve other facial muscles, leading to prominent eye blinks and grimacing. Tardive dyskinesia can proceed to involve spasms and dancelike movements of the shoulders, trunk, and limbs. The risk for tardive dyskinesia appears to increase with the dose of the medication and the length of time the child takes it. Generally there is minimal risk in a child who is receiving an agent for 1 month; however, children who are receiving these agents should be monitored for the development of abnormal muscle movements.

The treatment for tardive dyskinesia is usually removal of the antipsychotic drug, but this measure should not be taken lightly. Discontinuing the medication may actually worsen the tardive dyskinesia temporarily and is certainly likely to bring on the return of the behavioral/thought problems for which the medication has been prescribed. My patient, Jill, developed mild lip smacking while on 5 mg of Stelazine for her schizophrenia, and when we discontinued the medication over 2 weeks, Jill's tardive dyskinesia progressed to facial grimacing. The grimacing and lip smacking improved over the next 2 months, but stopping the antipsychotic medication had the predictable result of bringing back very disabling auditory hallucinations—voices the teenager heard telling her to harm herself. I am happy to report that she is now doing better on Risperdal. Pharmacological treatments may help reduce tardive dyskinesia. To date these drugs include many of the same agents used in adult neurology for the amelioration of Parkinson's disease. In addition, recent interest in the use of vitamin E has arisen, to possibly prevent tardive dyskinesia.

In any case, tardive dyskinesia should be distinguished from the more common, generally benign withdrawal spasms associated with the abrupt cessation of antipsychotic drugs that tend to subside without treatment after days to weeks of drug discontinuation. In children with mental retardation and pervasive developmental disorders, tardive dyskinesia should be differentiated from the commonly occurring stereotypies such as head banging or rocking.

---

stereotypies: Repetitive movements such as head banging or rocking.

THE ATYPICAL ANTIPSYCHOTICS

The newer generation of antipsychotics—Risperdal, Seroquel, Zyprexa, Geodon, and Abilify, and to a lesser extent Clozaril—are increasingly being used as first-line drugs of choice because side effects are less common, and they improve all aspects of psychosis. Symptoms such as withdrawal, loss of interest, ambivalence, and flattening of mood respond to these new antipsychotics. Like the traditional antipsychotics, they affect the dopamine system but appear to influence different subsets of dopamine and serotonin receptors. These newer drugs are being used for psychosis, marked mood swings, and severe tics/Tourette's disorder. Clozaril continues to be a highly effective agent reserved for treatment-refractory children and adolescents due to its intense monitoring requirements.

Dosing is based on their potency. Risperdal is the most potent of the agents. Therefore, the usual daily dose is lower and spans from 0.5 daily to 2 mg three times a day. Zyprexa is considered a middle-potency agent and is commonly dosed between 5 and 20 mg daily in children and adolescents. Seroquel and Clozaril are low-potency agents, and dosing ranges from 100 to 600 mg daily. It may take from 1 week to 3 months to see the full effectiveness of these agents, particularly Clozaril. Abilify and Geodon are considered midpotency drugs. Dosing of Geodon is 40–160 mg per day, and Abilify 5–30 mg per day in children.

Side effects of Risperdal, Zyprexa, and Seroquel appear similar to those of the traditional antipsychotics, but the rate of side effects and the risk for long-term tardive dyskinesia appear to be *substantially lower*. A transient increase in prolactin levels has been noted with Risperdal. This elevation is of unclear significance, and data suggest it is largely ameliorated after 6 months of treatment. Clozaril needs to be monitored very carefully since it has been associated with both a dangerous drop in blood cell production and severe seizures. Currently, weekly blood monitoring is necessary for Clozaril to be prescribed. The other agents do not require blood monitoring. In rare cases, a physician may request an EKG or an eye examination (Seroquel only). Because of weight gain associated with these medicines, attention to diet is imperative. In more extreme cases, adding Topamax (topiramate—50 mg twice a day) can be helpful in losing weight or keeping weight gain to a minimum.

Probably the most problematic long-term effects of any of the newest medications used to treat psychiatric disorders in children will be associated with the atypical antipsychotics, particularly Zyprexa and, to a lesser extent, Risperdal—largely because of their effects on increasing weight and potential effects on metabolism (concerns remain about a link between diabetes and the chronic use of atypical antipsychotics).

It is unclear that Seroquel or Geodon has these problems, and one of the very newest and very effective antipsychotics, Abilify (aripiprazole) while not increasing weight and being well tolerated, seems to cause a lot of motor spasms (dystonias) that *may* translate into a higher risk for tardive dyskinesia (irreversible motor writhing/twitches/spasms) with chronic use.

USE OF ANTIPSYCHOTICS

Over the past few years, clinicians tend to employ the atypical anti-psychotics as first-line agents for the treatment of children and adolescents who have severe disruptive disorders, self-injurious behavior, and bipolar disorder.

In children, hallucinations frequently occur with a mood disorder. In these cases, specific treatments for the mood disorder are crucial. It is not uncommon to place a child on lithium for bipolar disorder and Risperdal for the hallucinations. In cases where a child has disturbances in thought process along with severe agitation or anxiety, anxiety-breaking medications (benzodiazepines), such as lorazepam (Ativan) and clonazepam (Klonopin), can help and may also lead to the use of lower doses of antipsychotics. When single agents don't help, or in complicated cases, some children may require two medications: a mood-stabilizing agent such as lithium, Tegretol, or Depakote and an antipsychotic agent such as Risperdal, Seroquel, and Abilify. In these complicated cases, children may be receiving medications two or three times a day to the tune of eight tablets of medication daily.

The thought of combining agents can be uncomfortable to your child, family, and doctor, but it is often necessary. Twelve-year-old Jon had marked mood swings, irritability, anger outbursts, and the recent onset of hearing voices telling him to harm others and paranoia. Trilafon at 8 mg twice a day markedly reduced the hallucinations and paranoia, but he developed muscular spasms requiring Congentin. Jon's mood finally stabilized after he was placed on Tegretol 400 mg twice daily and Neurontin 300 mg twice daily. Jon tolerated the combination well despite receiving ten tablets of four different medications daily. Attempts to reduce the medications over the ensuing year resulted in recurrence of the moodiness and hallucinations.

CHAPTER 18

MEDICATIONS FOR SLEEP, BEDWETTING, AND OTHER PROBLEMS

A myriad of medications are used to treat problems that do not fall under the heading of emotional or behavioral problems yet often affect children with psychiatric disorders. These drugs come from different families and typically have more than one use. Clonidine, for one, is a blood pressure-lowering agent that is also useful for ADHD and, because of its sedative properties, for children who have trouble sleeping. Benadryl, for another, is used to relieve allergies but also serves as a sleep aid.

BENADRYL

Benadryl (diphenhydramine) is an antihistamine used commonly in all age groups for seasonal allergies, medication allergies, nonspecific rashes, and itching. Probably every family should keep a small quantity of Benadryl in the medicine cabinet. Because of its sedative properties, Benadryl can be very useful for assisting with children who are out of control and those with occasional sleep problems. Benadryl can also be beneficial in treating reactions to medications such as skin rashes and muscular spasms.

Benadryl has a very good track record in children and adolescents and is available in capsules, tablets, liquid (the preferable form because it works faster), and a better-tasting pediatric form. Typical dosing of full-strength Benadryl is 12.5 mg (½ teaspoon) for very young children, up to 50 mg for older children. Benadryl usually works within 30 minutes, and its effectiveness may last up to 8 hours. Its major side effects are short term and include sedation, morning drowsiness (if used at night), confusion at higher doses, and dry mouth. Benadryl probably should not be used long term since children rapidly develop tolerance to the sleep-inducing characteristics of the medication.

MELATONIN

Melatonin, a naturally occurring hormone related to sleep cycles in humans, has also been used in the treatment of sleep problems. During dark phases of the day, when most people are sleeping, melatonin levels naturally rise in the brain. Conversely, during daylight, melatonin levels diminish. Therefore introducing a "natural" compound around the hour of sleep is thought to induce a more natural sleep.

Some parents and one study have indicated that this agent helps children with a sleep disturbance (usually falling asleep) "relax" and fall asleep naturally. Controlled studies in children suggest that doses of 0.5 mg of melatonin capsules at bedtime are helpful and safe. Melatonin appears helpful for sleep disturbances related to psychiatric disorders as well as medications (e.g., stimulants). Side effects are not well studied in children but include morning sedation and changes in dream activity. Unlike some of the sleeping medications used in adults, because of its chemical nature, this drug does not appear to have significant addiction potential. No significant interactions between melatonin and psychotropic agents have been reported.

ANTIDIURETIC HORMONE DESMOPRESSIN

Children with bedwetting or enuresis not caused by a medical condition usually respond to nonpharmacological therapies. These treatments, including behavior modification and psychotherapy, should be considered first. Within the past 5 years, a synthetic form of a naturally occurring hormone called *antidiuretic hormone* has been used increasingly for bedwetting. This agent, called *desmopressin (ddAVP}*, comes in both a nose spray and a tablet form and is quite expensive.

Desmopressin safely and effectively suppresses urine production, generally for 7–10 hours. It is useful for children who want to sleep over at a friend's house or go to an overnight summer camp. Daily doses are one

(10 mg) to two sprays in each nostril prior to bedtime. Since bedwetting generally disappears with age, ddAVP therapy should not be continued indefinitely, although when used long term, it has been shown to be safe. Side effects are minimal and have been related to the more popular nasal spray, namely congestion and irritation inside the nose.

NALTREXONE

Naltrexone (Trexane or Rivea) appears helpful for two very different conditions: (1) the treatment of self-abuse such as self-mutilation and head banging; and (2) treatment of excessive alcohol intake in adolescents and adults. It appears that the drug naltrexone may work by blocking the effect of the natural opioid system in the brain called the *endorphin system;* it is a potent, long-acting agent that partially blocks the opioid, or natural pain relief, system of the brain. In both children with pervasive developmental disorders and those with self-abuse, the drug is used in daily doses of 25–150 mg daily. It appears that similar dosing may be necessary to reduce alcohol consumption, although at the time of this writing it has not been studied formally in adolescents. Although it is relatively free of serious adverse effects, there have been some rare reports of liver problems in adults, the majority of whom had preexisting liver problems, generally from alcoholism.

APPENDIX

Representative Medication Preparations and Sizes Used for the Treatment of Childhood Emotional and Behavioral Disorders

Medication		Sizes and preparation
Generic name	Brand name	
Stimulants		
Methylphenidate	Ritalin	5, 10, 20 mg; tablets
	Ritalin LA*	20, 30, 40 mg; capsules
	Methylin	20 mg; sustained-release tablets
	Focalin	2.5, 5, 10 mg; tablets
	Concerta*	18, 27, 36, 54 mg; capsules
	Metadate CD*	20 mg; capsules
Amphetamine compounds	Adderall	5, 10, 20, 30 mg; tablets
	Adderall XR*	5, 10, 15, 20, 25, 30 mg; capsules
Dextroamphetamine	Dexedrine	5, 10 mg; tablets
		5, 10, 15 mg; spansules
Magnesium pemoline	Cylert	18.75, 37.5, 75 mg; tablets
Nonstimulants (noradrenergic)		
Atomoxetine	Strattera	10, 18, 25, 40, 60 mg; capsules
Antihypertensives		
Clonidine	Catapres	0.1, 0.2., 0.3 mg; tablets
		1, 2, 3; skin patch
Guanfacine	Tenex	1 mg; tablet
Propranolol	Inderal	10, 20, 40, 60, 80 mg; tablets
		20, 60, 120 mg; sustained-release tablets
Nadolol	Corgard	20, 40, 80, 120, 160 mg; tablets

(cont.)

* Extended-release preparation (8- to 12-hour duration).

Antidepressants (selective serotonin reuptake inhibitors)

Fluoxetine	Prozac	10, 20, 60 mg; capsules 20 mg/tsp; suspension
Sertraline	Zoloft	50, 100 mg; tablets 20 mg/cc; suspension
Fluvoxamine	Luvox	50, 100 mg; tablets
Paroxetine	Paxil	10, 20, 30, 40 mg; tablets 20 mg/5 cc; suspension
Citalopram	Celexa	20, 40 mg; tablets
Escitalopram	Lexapro	10, 20 mg; tablets

Antidepressants (tricyclics)

Desipramine	Norpramin Pertofrane	10, 25, 50, 75, 100, 150 mg; tablets
Nortriptyline	Pamelor Vivactyl	10, 25, 50 mg; capsules 10 mg/tsp; oral suspension
Imipramine	Tofranil	10, 25, 50, 75, 100, 150 mg; tablets and capsules
Amitriptyline	Elavil	10, 25, 50, 75, 100, 150 mg; tablets
Protriptyline	Vivactyl	5, 10 mg; capsules
Maprotiline	Ludiomil	25, 50, 75 mg; tablets
Clomipramine	Anafranil	25, 50, 100 mg; tablets

Antidepressants (atypical)

Venlafaxine	Effexor	25, 37.5, 50, 75 mg; tablets 37.5, 75, 150 mg; extended-release tablets
Trazodone	Desyrel	50, 100, 150, 300 mg; tablets
Nefazodone	Serzone	50, 100, 200 mg; tablets
Bupropion	Wellbutrin	75, 100 mg; tablets 100, 150, 200 mg; sustained-release tablets 150, 300 mg; extended-release tablets

(cont.)

| Mirtazapine | Remeron | 15, 30 mg; tablets |
| Doxepin | Sinequan | 10, 25, 50, 75, 100, 150 mg; capsules
10 mg/cc; solution |

Monamine oxidase inhibitors
| Phenelzine | Nardil | 15 mg; tablets |
| Tranylcypromine | Parnate | 10 mg; tablets |

Antipsychotics (atypical)
Risperidone	Risperdal	0.25, 0.5, 1, 2, 3, mg; tablets
Olanzapine	Zyprexa	2.5, 5, 7.5, 10, 15 mg; tablets
Quetiapine	Seroquel	25, 100, 200 mg; tablets
Aripiprazole	Abilify	5, 10, 15, 20, 30 mg; tablets
Ziprasidone	Geodon	20, 40, 60, 80 mg; capsules
Clozapine	Clozaril	25, 50, 100 mg; tablets

Antipsychotics (high potency)
Haloperidol	Haldol	0.5, 1,2,5, 10, 20 mg; tablets 2 mg/ml; suspension
Pimozide	Orap	2 mg; tablet
Fluphenazine	Prolixin	2.5, 5, 10 mg; tablets 5 mg/ml; suspension

Antipsychotics (medium potency)
Trifluoperazine	Stelazine	1, 2, 5, 10 mg; tablets
Perphenazine	Trilafon	2, 4, 8, 16 mg; tablets
Thiothixene	Navane	2, 5, 10, 20 mg; tablets 5 mg/ml; suspension
Loxapine	Loxitane	5, 10, 25, 50 mg; tablets 5 mg/tsp; suspension

(cont.)

Antipsychotics (low potency)

Molindone   Moban   5, 10, 25, 50, 100 mg; tablets
                                      4 mg/tsp; suspension

Mesoridazine   Serentil   10, 25, 50, 100 mg; tablets
                                      25 mg/tsp; suspension

Thioridazine   Mellaril   10, 15, 25, 50, 100, 200 mg; tablets
                                      5, 6, 20 mg/tsp; suspension

Chlorpromazine   Thorazine   10, 25, 50, 100, 200 mg; tablets
                                      6, 20 mg/tsp; suspension

Mood stabilizers

Lithium salts   Lithobid,   150, 300, 450 mg; tablet
                     Lithonate,   8 mEq/tsp (= 300-mg tablet)
                     Lithotabs,
                     Eskalith,
                     Cibalith

Carbamazepine   Tegretol,   100, 200 mg; tablets
                     Carbachol   100 mg/tsp; suspension

Oxcarbazepine   Trileptal   150, 300, 600 mg; tablets

Valproic acid   Valproate,   125, 250, 500 mg; tablets and capsules
                     Depakote,   250 mg/tsp; suspension
                     Depakene
                     sprinkles

Gabapentin   Neurontin   100, 300, 400 mg; capsules
                                      400, 600, 800 mg; tablets

Lamotrigine   Lamictal   25, 100, 150, 200 mg; tablets

Topiramate   Topamax   25, 100, 200 mg; tablets

Tiagabine   Gabitril   4, 12, 16, 20 mg; tablets

(cont.)

Anxiety-breaking agents (anxiolytics)
Antihistamines

Diphenhydramine	Benadryl	25, 50 mg; tablets 25 mg/tsp; suspension
Hydroxyzine	Vistaril, Atarax	25, 50 mg; tablets 2 mg/tsp; suspension
Chlorpheniramine maleate	Chlor- Trimeton	2, 4, 8 mg; tablets

Benzodiazepines (partial list)

Clonazepam	Klonopin	0.5, 1, 2 mg; tablets
Alprazolam	Xanax	0.25, 0.5, 1 mg; tablets
Triazolam	Halcion	0.5, 1, 2 mg; tablets
Lorazepam	Ativan	0.5, 1 mg; tablets
Oxazepam	Serax	15, 30 mg; tablets
Diazepam	Valium	2, 5, 10 mg; tablets
Clorazepate	Tranxene	3.75, 7.5, 15 mg; capsules

Atypical

Buspirone	Buspar	5, 10, 15 mg; tablets
Zolpidem	Ambien	5, 10 mg; tablets
Zaleplon	Sonata	5, 10 mg; tablets

Example of a Completed Medication Log

Start date/ end date	Medication	Daily dose	Response	Side effect(s)	Comments
11/02–2/03	Ritalin	20 mg BID	Very good	Edginess	Good school performance
2/03–3/03	Concerta	54 mg	Very good	Edginess	Good school performance
2/03–4/03	Adderall XR	10–20 mg	Very good	Edginess Moodiness	Good school performance
4/03–7/03	Strattera	60 mg	Good	Tired	Good behavior, attention problems
7/03–	Strattera + Concerta	60 mg 54 mg	Excellent	None	Good school and behavior Improved mood

Medication Log

Start date/ end date	Medication	Daily dose	Response	Side effect(s)	Comments

RESOURCES

The following are organizations promoting mental health issues in children and adolescents.

GENERAL INFORMATION

American Academy of Child and Adolescent Psychiatry
3615 Wisconsin Avenue, NW
Washington, DC 20016-3007
Phone: 202-966-7300
Website: *www.aacap.org*

The largest organization of child and adolescent psychiatrists who practice, research, and teach about the myriad of mental health problems in youth. The organization has superb educational materials for families and extensive lists of local child psychiatrists available for care.

American Academy of Pediatrics
141 Northwest Point Boulevard
Elk Grove Village, IL 60007-1098
Phone: 847-434-4000
Website: *www.aap.org*

The largest national organization of pediatricians. The academy has many educational materials on a myriad of common child psychiatric disorders.

American International Health Alliance
1212 New York Avenue, NW, Suite 750
Washington, DC 20005
Phone: 202-789-1136
Fax: 202-789-1277
E-mail: webmaster@aiha.com
Website: *www.aiha.com*

American Psychiatric Association
1000 Wilson Boulevard, Suite 1825
Arlington, VA 22209-3901
Phone: 703-907-7300
Website: *www.psych.org*

A broad-based organization with 35,000 physican members—the oldest medical specialty organization in the United States—that publishes the *Diagnostic and Statistical Manual of Mental Disorders* and many other resources for mental health professionals, establishes psychiatric practice standards, advocates for mental health patients, provides voluminous public information, and supports education and research.

Brain Connections
Website: *neuro-www.mgh.harvard.edu/brainconnections.html*

A conglomeration of free and for-fee sources (conferences) of up-to-date information on a wide spectrum of mental health issues.

Federation of Families for Children's Mental Health
1101 King Street, Suite 420
Alexandria, VA 22314
Phone: 703-684-7710
Website: *www.ffcmh.org*

A broad-based organization run by parents who publish a newsletter and have regional meetings focused on children and adolescents with a myriad of psychiatric problems.

General Mental Health Sources on the Net
Website: *www.dana.org/dabi/brainconnections.html*

A very user-friendly and excellent source for accessing many other sites on the Web related to mental health (and other disabilities). Many of the resources listed in this section can be located using this site.

MIND (National Association for Mental Health United Kingdom)
Granta House, 15—19 Broadway
London E15 4BQ, United Kingdom
Phone: 44 (0)20 8519 2122
Website: *www.mind.org.uk*

The leading mental health charity in England and Wales provides links to numerous articles on children's mental health in the United Kingdom.

National Alliance for the Mentally Ill
Colonial Place Three
2107 Wilson Boulevard, Suite 300
Arlington, VA 22201-3042
Phone: 703-524-7600
Fax: 703-524-9094
TDD: 703-516-7227
Member services: 888-999-NAMI
Website: *www.nami.org*

A large mental health organization focused on all individuals with mental illness. This group provides an infrastructure for support groups, advocacy (local and national), and regional and national conferences. More recently, the NAMI has expanded to include child-based issues.

National Institute of Mental Health
NIMH Public Inquiries
6001 Executive Boulevard, Room 8184, MSC 9663
Bethesda, MD 20892-9663
Phone: 301-443-4513
Toll free: 866-615-NIMH (6464)
TTY: 301-443-8431; Fax: 301-443-4279
FAX 4U: 301-443-5158
E-mail: nimhinfo@nih.gov
Website: *www.nimh.nih.gov*

This subsection of the United States Public Health Service is the major government agency involved in the research of juvenile behavioral, emotional, and cognitive disorders. In addition to providing funding for a variety of research activity, the NIMH is involved in conferences and public policy.

National Mental Health Association
2001 North Beauregard Street, 12th floor
Alexandria, VA 22311
Main Switchboard: 703-684-7722
Toll free: 800-969-NMHA (6642)
TTY: 800-433-5959
Fax: 703-684-5968
Website: *www.nmha.org*

A large, client-oriented organization that disseminates information on all aspects of mental illness across the lifespan. Referrals of practitioners knowledgeable in the diagnosis and treatment of specific emotional, behavioral, and cognitive disorders as well as local support groups are available.

ANXIETY DISORDERS

Anxiety Disorders Association of America
8730 Georgia Avenue, Suite 600
Silver Spring, MD 20910
Phone: 240-485-1001
Website: *www.adaa.org*

By offering self-help tools, professional development resources, information on clinical trials, and access to legislative action events and partnerships, this national nonprofit organization promotes early diagnosis, treatment, and cure of anxiety disorders across the lifespan.

Freedom from Fear
308 Seaview Avenue
Staten Island, NY 10305
Phone: 718-351-1717
Fax: 718-667-8893
Website: *www.freedomfromfear.com*

A 20-year-old national nonprofit advocacy association dedicated to helping people with depressive and anxiety disorders. A main feature is its anxiety and depression screening program with free consultation with a mental health professional. Also up-to-date news coverage of related topics.

Selective Mutism Foundation
P.O. Box 13133
Sissonville, WV 25360-0133
Website: *www.selectivemutismfoundation.org*

A focused organization covering mutism in youth and adulthood. Referrals of prac-titioners knowledgeable in the diagnosis and treatment of mutism are available. For information, send a self-addressed envelope with two stamps.

ATTENTION-DEFICIT/HYPERACTIVITY DISORDER

Attention Deficit Disorder Association
P.O. Box 543
Pottstown, PA 19464
Phone: 484-945-2101
Website: *www.add.org*

A "hotline" focused on ADHD with phone numbers and locations of local support groups. In addition, this organization sponsors a yearly conference on ADHD.

Children and Adults with Attention-Deficit/Hyperactivity Disorder
8181 Professional Place, Suite 150
Landover, MD 20785
Toll free: 800-233-4050
Website: *www.chadd.org*

The largest of many organizations offering support and educational materials for children, adolescents, and adults with ADHD (and their families). A yearly confer-ence sponsored by CHADD is available providing a comprehensive understanding and update of ADHD. Referrals of local practitioners knowledgeable in the diagno-sis and treatment of ADHD as well as local support groups are available.

AUTISM/PERVASIVE DEVELOPMENTAL DISORDERS/ ASPERGER SYNDROME

Autism Research Institute
4182 Adams Avenue
San Diego, CA 92116
Fax: 619-563-6840
Website: *www.autism/com/ari*

More than 35 years old, this nonprofit organization is devoted mainly to conducting research into the causes of autism as well as methods for prevention, diagnosis, and treatment.

Autism Society of America
7910 Woodmont Avenue, Suite 300
Bethesda, MD 20814-3067
Toll free: 800-3AUTISM
Website: *www.autism-society.org*

A large organization offering support and educational materials for children, adolescents, and adults (and their families) with autism and related disorders including Asperger syndrome and pervasive developmental disorder. A yearly conference sponsored by the society is available providing a comprehensive understanding and update on autism and related disorders. Referrals of local practitioners knowledgeable in the diagnosis and treatment of autism as well as local support groups are available.

The National Autistic Society (United Kingdom)
393 City Road
London EC1V 1NG, United Kingdom
Phone: 44 (0)20 7833 2299
Fax: 44 (0)20 7833 9666
E-mail: nas@nas.org.uk
Website: *www.nas.org.uk/*

Provides information and services, from diagnosis to family support, on autism and Asperger syndrome in the United Kingdom. Lists fundraising events and provides access to a research database and a wealth of publications.

EATING DISORDERS

American Anorexia Bulimia Association, Inc.
165 West 46th Street, Suite 1108
New York, NY 10036
Phone: 212-575-6200
Website: *www.aabinc.org*

This organization provides referrals of local practitioners, groups, inpatient facilities with particular expertise in the diagnosis and treatment of eating disorders.

ANRED: Anorexia Nervosa and Related Eating Disorders, Inc.
P.O. Box 5102
Eugene, OR 97405
Phone: 541-344-1144
Toll free: 800-931-2237
Website: *www.anred.com*

A mainly educational organization with a newsletter and lists of local and regional educators in the disorder.

Eating Disorders Association (United Kingdom)
Windsor House, 1st Floor
103 Prince of Wales Road
Norwich NR1 1DW, United Kingdom
Phone: 44 (0)16 0362 1414
Helpline: 44 (0)84 5634 1414
Youth Helpline: 44 (0)84 5634 7650
E-mail: info@edauk.com
Webstite: *www.edauk.com*

A nonprofit organization aimed at providing information, help, and support for those with eating disorders, as well as raising standards of care and availability of treatment. Features a self-help network and wide range of resources for getting help.

Eating Disorders Resource Centre (Australia)
P.O. Box 138
Wilston, Queensland 4051, Australia
Phone: 61 (0)7 3352 6900
E-mail: eda.inc@uq.net.au
Website: *www.uq.net.au/eda/documents/start.html*

A nonprofit organization dedicated to improving intervention, education, and support for those with eating disorders as well as to improving awareness and promoting prevention.

National Eating Disorders Association
603 Stewart Street, Suite 803
Seattle, WA 98101
Phone: 206-382-3587
Toll free: 800-931-2237
Website: *www.nationaleatingdisorders.org*

The largest nonprofit organization in the United States dedicated to preventing eating disorders. Develops prevention programs, publishes and distributes educational materials, and operates the nation's first toll-free eating disorders information and referral helpline.

MOOD DISORDERS

Child and Adolescent Bipolar Foundation
1187 Wilmette Avenue
P. M. Box #331
Wilmette, IL 60091
Phone: 847-256-8525
Fax: 847-920-9498
Website: *www.bpkids.org*

An excellent parent support group that has a very user-friendly website. This group provides excellent education about bipolar disorder and is a well-regarded advocate for bipolar disorder in the scientific and political domains.

Depression and Bipolar Support Alliance
730 North Franklin Street, Suite 501
Chicago, IL 60610-7204
Phone: 312-642-0049
Toll free: 800-826-3632
Website: *www.ndmda.org*

A national organization dedicated to improving the lives of those with mood disorders, with over 1,000 support groups run by chapters.

Depression and Related Affective Disorders Association
2330 West Joppa Road, Suite 100
Lutherville, MD 21093
Phone: 410-583-2919
Website: *www.drada.org*

A community organization designed to assist self-help groups, provide education and information, and lend support to research programs related to depression and bipolar disorder.

Depression Alliance (United Kingdom)
35 Westminster Bridge Road
London SE1 7JB, United Kingdom
Phone: 44 (0)20 7633 0557
Fax: 44 (0)20 7633 0559
Website: *www.depressionalliance.org/*

The United Kingdom's leading association for depression offers a wealth of information about symptoms and treatment as well as the alliance's campaigns and access to support groups.

Manic Depression Fellowship (United Kingdom)
Castle Works 21 St. Georges Road
London SE1 6ES, United Kingdom
National advice line: 44(0)208 7793 2600
Scotland advice line: 44(0)141 400 1867
Wales advice line: 44(0)1633 244 244
Website: *www.mdf.org.uk/*

A 20-year-old nonprofit organization devoted to improving the lives of people with bipolar disorder by making available self-help groups, publications, a legal advice hotline, and a self-management training program.

National Depressive and Manic–Depressive Association
730 North Franklin Street, Suite 501
Chicago, IL 60610-7204
Phone: 312-642-0049
Fax: 312-642-7243
Toll free: 800-826-3632
E-mail: questions@ndmda.org
Website: *www.ndmda.org*

Offering 275 chapters and support groups, NDMDA is the nation's largest patient-run, illness-specific organization. Its mission is to educate the public about depressive and manic–depressive illnesses; to foster self-help; to eliminate discrimination and stigma; to improve access to care; and to advocate for research. Callers will not receive advice about medications or physician referrals.

OBSESSIVE–COMPULSIVE DISORDER
AND TOURETTE'S DISORDER

Obsessive–Compulsive Foundation
676 State St.
New Haven, CT 06511
Phone: 203-401-2070
Website: *www.ocfoundation.org*

A 10,000-member international nonprofit organization aimed at educating the public and professionals, assisting patients with obsessive–compulsive disorder and their families, and supporting research. Publishes newsletters, holds annual conferences, maintains a provider list of specialists, operates a training institute for practitioners, and organizes and promotes support groups.

Obsessive Compulsive Information Center
Dean Foundation for Health and Education
8000 Excelsior Drive, Suite 302
Madison, WI 53717
Phone: 608-836-8070
Website: *www.miminc.org*

A resource for information on obsessive–compulsive disorder and related disorders operated under the aegis of the Madison Institute of Medicine that provides not only 19,000 references on everything from diagnosis to treatment but patient guides and information packets.

National Institute of Neurological Disorders and Stroke
NIH Neurological Institute
P.O. Box 5801
Bethesda, MD 20825
Phone: 301-496-5751
Toll free: 800-352-9424
Website: *www.ninds.nih.gov*

A government-funded resource on neurologically related disorders that overlap with psychiatric disorders.

Tourette Syndrome Association, Inc.
42-40 Bell Boulevard
Bayside, NY 11361-2820
Phone: 718-224-2999
Website: *www.tsa-usa.org*

This organization is for individuals with Tourette's disorder and their families and is well known for its support and dissemination of research on Tourette's and related disorders. A thoughtful newsletter encompasses recent findings and ongoing research in the area of Tourette's disorder. Referrals of local practitioners knowledgeable in the diagnosis and treatment of Tourette's disorder as well as local support groups are available.

Trichotillomania Learning Center
303 Potrero Street #51
Santa Cruz, CA 95060
Phone: 408-457-1004
Website: *www.trich.org*

PSYCHOSIS

International Early Psychosis Association (Australia)
Locked Bag 10
Parkville, Victoria 3052, Australia
Phone: 61 (0)3 9342 2837
Fax: 61 (0)3 9342 2941
Website: *www.iepa.org.au*

This international organization based in Australia provides a forum for international collaboration and communication on psychosis in young people by facilitating research and optimal diagnostic and treatment practices, arranging conferences, and advocating public policies that will improve services to patients.

National Alliance for Research on Schizophrenia and Depression
60 Cutter Mill Road, Suite 404
Great Neck, NY 11021
Phone: 516-829-0091
Toll free: 800-829-8289
Fax: 516-487-6930
Website: *www.narsad.org*

Mainly research-based, this organization sponsors small grants for studies related to schizophrenia and depression. Members receive an acclaimed newsletter with timely findings on mental health.

National Schizophrenic Fellowship (Rethink) (United Kingdom)
Inquiries: 44 (0)84 5456 0455
E-mail: info@rethink.org
National advice hotline: 44 (0)20 8974 6814
Website: *www.rethink.org*

The United Kingdom's largest nonprofit organization devoted to severe mental
illness provides a wide range of community services aimed at allowing patients to
take greater control of their lives and also advocates for policies and practices that
will support that goal and the goals of increasing awareness and reducing stigma.

SLEEP DISORDERS

American Academy of Sleep Medicine
One Westbrook Corporate Center, Suite 920
Westchester, IL 60154
Phone: 708-492-0930
Fax: 708-492-0943
Website: *www.aasmnet.org*

This national professional organization provides patient resources, from a sleep
quiz to locations of sleep centers across the United States to links to related sites.

American Insomnia Association
One Westbrook Corporate Center, Suite 920
Westchester, IL 60154
Phone: 708-492-0930
Fax: 708-492-0943
Website: *www.americaninsomniaassociation.org*

A patient-based organization that provides a variety of information and sources of
information on medications and other treatment options for insomnia.

National Center on Sleep Disorders Research
National Heart, Lung, and Blood Institute
National Institutes of Health
6705 Rockledge Drive
One Rockledge Centre, Suite 6022
Bethesda, MD 20892-7993
Phone: 301-435-0199
Fax: 301-480-3451
Website: *www.nhlbi.nih.gov/about/ncsdr/*

A government-funded organization that has information available about sleep-related problems.

SUBSTANCE ABUSE

Canadian Centre on Substance Abuse
75 Albert Street, Suite 300
Ottawa ON K1P 5E7, Canada
Phone: 613-235-4048
Fax: 613-235-8101
Website: *www.ccsa.ca*

Helplines, toolkits, directories, news archives, informational databases, prevention activities, and links to other sites from Canada's 15-year-old national addictions agency.

National Addiction Centre (United Kingdom)
Institute of Psychiatry
King's College London
De Crespigny Park SE5 8AF, United Kingdom
Phone: 44 (0)20 7848 0811
E-mail: D.Ball@iop.bpmf.ac.uk
Website: *www.iop.kcl.ac.uk/IoP/Deaprtments/PsychMed/NAC/index.shtml*

From the website: "A network of clinicians, researchers and clinical teachers sharing a commitment to excellence in work directed at the prevention and treatment of substance misuse, and to the support and strengthening of national and international endeavours in this field."

National Institute on Drug Abuse
6001 Executive Boulevard
Bethesda, MD 20892-9561
Toll free: 800-729-6686 (for information on drug abuse); 800-662-4357 (for information on counselors, treatment facilities)
Website: *www.nida.nih.gov*

National Institute on Alcohol Abuse and Alcoholism
6000 Executive Boulevard, Willco Building
Bethesda, MD 20892-7003
Website: *www.niaaa.nih.gov*

These subsections of the United States Public Health Service are the major government agencies involved in the research of juvenile and adult drug and alcohol use, misuse, abuse, and dependence. In addition to providing funding for a variety of research activities, NIDA and NIAAA are involved in conferences and public policy. NIDA has an incredibly informative and user-friendly website—one of the best I have seen.

Network of Alcohol/Drug Agencies, Australia
295 Cleveland Street
Surry Hills 2010, New South Wales, Australia
Phone: 61(02) 9698 8669
Fax: 61(02) 9690 0727
E-mail: admin@nada.org.au
Website: *www.nada.org.au*

The principal organization for the alcohol and drug nongovernment sector throughout New South Wales, funded by NSW Health, with a membership made up of over 100 agencies. A good source of information on policy issues and advocacy.

PHARMACEUTICAL COMPANIES

Most of the medications listed in this book have a dedicated website sponsored by the respective pharmaceutical company. Many of these are accessed by typing the medication (usually the brand name) into your search engine or by using *www.[drugname].com*. These sites often contain detailed information about side effects and FDA-approved use of these compounds. Some of the websites have links to other websites of interest, many of which are maintained by nonprofit organizations.

BIBLIOGRAPHY

GENERAL

Baldessarini, R. J. (1996). *Chemotherapy in Psychiatry*. Harvard University Press, Cambridge, MA.

Green, W. H. (1991). *Child and Adolescent Clinical Psychopharmacology*. Williams & Wilkins, Baltimore.

Greene, R. W. (1998). *The Explosive Child: A New Approach for Understanding and Parenting Easily Frustrated, "Chronically Inflexible" Children*. HarperCollins, New York.

Koplewicz, H. (1996). *It's Nobody's Fault*. Times Books, New York.

Martin A., Scahhill, L., Charney, D., & Leckman, J. (2003). *Pediatric Psychopharmacology*, Oxford University Press, New York.

Plizka, S. R. (2003). *Neuroscience for the Mental Health Clinician*. Guilford Press, New York.

Popper, C. (1987). *Psychiatric Pharmacosciences of Children and Adolescents*. American Psychiatric Press, Washington, DC.

Ratey, J. J. (1991). *Mental Retardation: Developing Pharmacotherapies (Progress in Psychiatry,* Vol. 32). American Psychiatric Press, Washington, DC.

Riddle, M., ed. (1995). *Pediatric Psychopharmacology (Child and Adolescent Clinics of North America,* Vols. 1 & 2). Saunders, Philadelphia.

Roberts, R., Attkisson, C., & Rosenblatt, A. (1998). Prevalence of psychopathology among children and adolescents. *American Journal of Psychiatry, 155,* 715–725.

Rosenberg, D. R., Hottum, J., & Gershon, S. (1994). *Pharmacotherapy for Child and Adolescent Psychiatric Disorders*. Brunner/Mazel, New York.

Rutter, M., & Rutter, M. (1993). *Developing Minds*. HarperCollins, New York.

Rutter M., Taylor, E., & Hersov, L. (1994). *Child and Adolescent Psychiatry: Modern Approaches*. Plenum, New York.

Stahl, S. M. (2000). *Essential Psychopharmacology: Neuroscientific Basis and Practical Applications*. Cambridge University Press, Cambridge, England.

Swedo, S., & Leonard, H. (1996). *It's Not All in Your Head.* HarperCollins, San Francisco.

Weiner, J., ed. (2004). *Textbook of Child and Adolescent Psychiatry* (3rd ed.). American Psychiatric Press, Washington, DC.

Wilens, T., Spencer, T., Biederman, J., & Linehan, C. (1996). Child and adolescent psychopharmacology. In R. Michels, ed., *Psychiatry* (pp. 1–26). Lippincott, Washington, DC.

ANXIETY DISORDERS

Barlow, D. (2002). *Anxiety and Its Disorders* (2nd ed.). Guilford Press, New York.

Beck, A. (1990). *Anxiety Disorders and Phobias: A Cognitive Perspective* (rep. ed.). Basic Books, New York.

Bernstein, G., Borchardt, C., & Perwein, A. (1996). Anxiety disorders in children and adolescents: A review of the past 10 years. *Journal of the American Academy of Child and Adolescent Psychiatry, 35,* 1110–1119.

Birmaher, B., Waterman, G. S., Ryan, N., Cully, M., Balach, L., Ingram, J., & Brodsky, M. (1994). Fluoxetine for childhood anxiety disorders. *Journal of the American Academy of Child and Adolescent Psychiatry, 33,* 993–999.

Clark, D. B., Smith, M. G., Neighbors, B. D., Skerlec, L. M., & Randall, J. (1994). Anxiety disorders in adolescence: Characteristics, prevalence, and comorbidities. *Clinical Psychology Review, 14*(2), 113–137.

Davidson, J. (2003). *The Anxiety Book: Developing Strength in the Face of Fear.* Riverhead Books, New York.

Klein, R. G., & Last, C. G. (1989). Anxiety disorders in children. In A. Kazdin, ed., *Developmental Clinical Psychology and Psychiatry* (Vol. 20). Sage, Newbury Park, CA.

Last, C. G., Perrin, S., Hersen, M., & Kazdin, A. E. (1996). A prospective study of childhood anxiety disorders. *Journal of the American Academy of Child and Adolescent Psychiatry, 35*(11), 1502–1510.

Pine, D. S. (2002). Treating children and adolescents with selective serotonin reuptake inhibitors: How long is appropriate? *Journal of Child and Adolescent Psychopharmacology, 12,*(3), 189–203.

Pine, D. S., & Grun, J. (1999). Childhood anxiety: Integrating developmental psychopathology and affective neuroscience. *Journal of Child and Adolescent Psychopharmacology, 9*(1), 1–12.

Swedo, S. E., Fleeter, J. D., Richter, D. M., Hoffman, C. L., Allen, A. J., Hamburger, S. D., Turner, E. H., Yamada, E. M., & Rosenthal, N. E. (1995). Rates of seasonal affective disorder in children and adolescents. *American Journal of Psychiatry, 152,* 1016–1019.

Bernstein, G. A., Borchardt, C. M., Perwien, A. R., Crosby, R. D., Kushner, M. G., Thuras, P. D., & Last, C. G. (2000). Imipramine plus cognitive-behavioral therapy in the treatment of school refusal. *Journal of the American Academy of Child and Adolescent Psychiatry, 39*(3), 276–283.

Walkup, J., Labellarte, M. J., Riddle, M., Pine, D. S., Greenhill, L., Klein, R., Davies, M., Sweeney, M., Abikoff, H., Hack, S., Klee, B., McCracken, J. T., Bergman, L., Piacentini, J., March, J., Compton, S., Robinson, J., O'Hara, T., Baker, S., Vitiello, B., Ritz, L., Roper, M., & The Research Unit on Pediatric Psychopharmacology Anxiety Study Group. (2001). Fluvoxamine for the treatment of anxiety disorders in children and adolescents. The Research Unit on Pediatric Psychopharmacology Anxiety Study Group. *New England Journal of Medicine, 344*(17), 1279–1285.

ATTENTION–DEFICIT/HYPERACTIVITY DISORDER

Barkley, R. A. (1997). *ADHD and the Nature of Self-Control.* Guilford Press, New York.

Barkley, R. A. (1998). *Attention-Deficit Hyperactivity Disorder: A Handbook for Diagnosis and Treatment* (2nd ed.). Guilford Press, New York.

Barkley, R. A., Edwards, G., Laneri, M., Fletcher, K., & Metevia, L. (2001). Executive functioning, temporal discounting, and sense of time in adolescents with attention deficit hyperactivity disorder (ADHD) and oppositional defiant disorder (ODD). *Journal of Abnormal Child Psychology, 29*(6), 541–555.

Barkley, R. A., Murphy, K. R., Dupaul, G. I., & Bush, T. (2002). Driving in young adults with attention deficit hyperactivity disorder: knowledge, performance, adverse outcomes, and the role of executive functioning. *Journal of the International Neuropsychology Society, 8*(5), 655–672.

Biederman, J., Faraone, S. V., & Mick, E. (2000). Age dependent decline of ADHD symptoms revisited: Impact of remission definition and symptom subtype. *American Journal of Psychiatry, 157, 816–817.*

Biederman, J., & Spencer, T. (1999). Attention deficit hyperactivity disorder (ADHD) as a noradrenergic disorder. *Biological Psychiatry, 46*(9), 1234–1242.

Biederman, J., Baldessarini, R. J., Wright, V., Knee, D., & Harmatz, J. S. (1989). A double-blind placebo controlled study of despramine in the treatment of ADD: I. Efficacy. *Journal of the American Academy of Child and Adolescent Psychiatry, 28, 777–784.*

Biederman, J., Newcorn, J., & Sprich, S. (1991). Comorbidity of attention deficit hyperactivity disorder with conduct, depressive, anxiety, and other disorders. *American Journal of Psychiatry, 148, 564–577.*

Brown, T. (1999). *Subtypes of Attention Deficit Disorders in Children, Adolescents, and Adults.* American Psychiatric Press, Washington, DC.

Conners, C., & Jett, J. (1999). *Attention Deficit Hyperactivity Disorder (in Adults and Children): The Latest Assessment and Treatment Strategies.* Compact Clinicals, Salt Lake City.

Connor, D. (1993). Beta-blockers for aggression: The pediatric experience. *Journal of Child and Adolescent Psychopharmacology, 3,* 99–114.

Goldman, L., Genel, M., Bezman, R., & Slanetz, P. (1998). Diagnosis and treatment of attention-deficit/hyperactivity disorder in children and adolescents. *Journal of the American Medical Association, 279,* 1100–1107.

Greenhill, L. L., & Osman, B. B. (1991). *Ritalin: Theory and Patient Management.* Mary Ann Liebert, New York.

Greenhill, L., & Osman, B., eds. (1999). *Ritalin: Theory and Practice.* Mary Ann Liebert, New York.

Greenhill, L. L., Pliszka, S., Dulcan, M. K., Bernet, W., Arnold, V., Beitchman, J., Benson, R. S., Bukstein, O., Kinlan, J., McClellan, J., Rue, D., Shaw, J. A., & Stock, S. (2002). Practice parameter for the use of stimulant medications in the treatment of children, adolescents, and adults. *Journal of the American Academy of Child and Adolescent Psychiatry, 41*(2; Suppl.), 26S–49S.

Hunt, R. D., Arnsten, A. F., & Asbell, M. D. (1995). An open trial of guanfacine in the treatment of attention deficit hyperactivity disorder. *Journal of the American Academy of Child and Adolescent Psychiatry, 34,* 50–54.

Hunt, R. D., Minderaa, R. B., & Cohen, D. J (1985). Clonidine benefits children with attention deficit disorder and hyperactivity: Report of a double-blind placebo-crossover therapeutic trial. *Journal of the American Academy of Child and Adolescent Psychiatry, 24,* 617–629.

Kolberg J., & Nadeau, K. (2002). *ADD-Friendly Ways to Organize Your Life.* Brunner-Routledge, New York.

Mannuzza, S., Klein, R. G., Bessler, A., Malloy, P., & LaPadula, M. (1993). Adult outcome of hyperactive boys: Educational achievement, occupational rank, and psychiatric status. *Archives of General Psychiatry, 50,* 565–576.

Mannuzza, S., Klein, R. G., Bonagura, N., Malloy, P., Giampino, T. L., & Addalli, K. A. (1991). Hyperactive boys almost grown up: V. Replication of psychiatric status. *Archives of General Psychiatry, 48,* 77–83.

MTA Cooperative Group. (1999). A 14-month randomized clinical trial of treatment strategies for attention-deficit/hyperactivity disorder. *Archives of General Psychiatry, 56,* 1073–1086.

Pelham, W. E., Greenslade, K. E., Vodde-Hamilton, M., Murphy, D. A., Greenstein, J. J., Gnagy, E. M., Guthrie, K. J., Hoover, M. D., & Dahl, R. E. (1990). Relative efficacy of long-acting stimulants on children with attention deficit-hyperactivity disorder: A comparison of standard methylphenidate, sustained-release methylphenidate, sustained-release dextroamphetamine, and pemoline. *Pediatrics, 86,* 226–237.

Safer, D. J., & Zito, J. M. (1996). Increased methylphenidate usage for ADHD. *Pediatrics, 98,* 1084–1088.

Safer, D., & Zito, J. (1999). Pharmacoepidemiology of methylphenidate and other stimulants for the treatment of ADHD. In L. Greenhill & B. Osman, eds., *Ritalin: Theory and Practice* (pp. 7–26). Mary Ann Liebert, New York.

Safer, D. J., & Allen, R. P. (1989). Absence of tolerance to the behavioral effects of methylphenidate in hyperactive and inattentive children. *Journal of Pediatrics, 115*(6), 1003–1008.

Spencer, T. J., Biederman, J., Wilens, T. E., Harding, M., O'Donnell, D., & Griffin, S. (1996). Pharmacotherapy of ADHD across the lifecycle: A literature review. *Journal of the American Academy of Child and Adolescent Psychiatry, 35,* 409–432.

Spencer, T., Biederman, J., Harding, M., O'Donnell, D., Faraone, S., & Wilens, T. (1996). Growth deficits in ADHD children revisited: Evidence for disorder-associated growth delays? *Journal of the American Academy of Child and Adolescent Psychiatry, 35,* 1460–1469.

Spencer, T., Biederman, J., & Wilens, T. (1998). Pharmacotherapy of attention-deficit/hyperactivity disorder: A life span perspective. In L. Dickstein, M. Riba, & J. Oldham, eds., *Review of Psychiatry* (Vol. IV, pp. 87–127). American Psychiatric Press, Washington, DC.

Spencer, T. J., Biederman, J., Faraone, S., Mick, E., Coffey, B., Geller, D., Kagan, J., Bearman, S. K., & Wilens, T. (2001). Impact of tic disorders on ADHD outcome across the life cycle: Findings from a large group of adults with and without ADHD. *American Journal of Psychiatry, 158*(4), 611–617.

Swanson, J. M., McBurnett, K., Christian, D. L., & Wigal, T. (1995). Stimulant medications and the treatment of children with ADHD. *Advances in Clinical Child Psychology, 17,* 265–322.

Swanson, J., Gupta, S., Guinta, D., Flynn, D., Agler, D., Lerner, M., Williams, L., Shoulson, I., & Wigal, S. (1992). Acute tolerance to methylphenidate in the treatment of attention deficit hyperactivity disorder in children. *Clinical Pharmacological Therapy, 66*(3), 295–305.

Swanson, J., Lerner, M., Gupta, S., Shoulson, I., & Wigal, S. (2003). Development of a new once-a-day formulation of methylphenidate for the treatment of ADHD: Proof of concept and proof of product studies. *Archives of General Psychiatry, 60*(2), 204–211.

Umansky, W. (2003). *AD/HD: Helping Your Child: A Comprehensive Program to Treat Attention Deficit/Hyperactivity Disorders at Home and in School.* Warner Books, New York.

Weiss, G., & Hechtman, L. T. (1986). *Hyperactive Children Grown Up.* The Guilford Press, New York.

Weiss, G. (1992). *Attention-Deficit Hyperactivity Disorder.* Saunders, Philadelphia.

Weiss, G., & Hechtman, L. T. (1993). *Hyperactive Children Grown Up* (2nd ed.). Guilford Press, New York.

Wender, P. (1987). *The Hyperactive Child, Adolescent, and Adult: Attention Deficit Disorder through the Lifespan.* Oxford University Press, New York.

Werry, J., ed. (1994). *Pharmacotherapy of Disruptive Behavior Disorders (Child and Adolescent Psychiatric Clinics of North America,* Vol. 3). Saunders, Philadelphia.

Wilens, T. E., & Biederman, J. (1992). The stimulants. In D. Shaffer, ed., *Psychiatric Clinics of North America* (pp. 191–222). Saunders, Philadelphia.

Wilens, T., Biederman, J., & Spencer, T. (2002). Attention Deficit Hyperactivity Disorder. In C. T. Caskey, ed., *Annual Review of Medicine, 53,* 113–131.

Wilens, T., Faraone, S., Biederman, J., & Gunawardene, S. (2003). Does stimulant therapy of ADHD beget later substance abuse: A metanalytic review of the literature. *Pediatrics, 11*(1), 179–185.

Wolraich, M. L., Lindgren, S. D., Stumbo, P. J., Stegink, L. D., Appelbaum, M. I., & Kiritsy, M. C. (1994). Effects of diets high in sucrose or aspartame on the behavior and cognitive performance of children. *New England Journal of Medicine, 330,* 301–307.

Zametkin, A., & Liotta, W. (1998). The neurobiology of attention-deficit/hyperactivity disorder. *Journal of Clinical Psychiatry, 59*(1), 7–23.

AUTISM/PERVASIVE DEVELOPMENTAL DISORDER

Aman, M. G., De Smedt, G., Derivan, A., Lyons, B., & Findling, R. L. (2002). Double-blind, placebo-controlled study of risperidone for the treatment of disruptive behaviors in children with subaverage intelligence. *American Journal of Psychiatry, 159*(8), 1337–1346.

Attwood, T. (1998). *Asperger's Syndrome: A Guide for Parents and Professionals.* Jessica Kinsley, Philadelphia.

Campbell, M., Small, A., & Green, W. (1984). Behavioral efficacy of haloperidol and lithium carbonate. *Archives of General Psychiatry, 41,* 650–656.

Campbell, M. (1984). Fenfluramine treatment of autism. *Journal of Child Psychology and Psychiatry and Allied Disciplines, 29,* 1–10.

Feldman, H. M., Kolmen, B. K., & Gonzaga, A. M. (1999). Naltrexone and communication skills in young children with autism. (1999). *Journal of the American Academy of Child and Adolescent Psychiatry, 38*(5), 587–593.

Gross, J. (2003, Nov. 19). Government mapping out a strategy to fight autism, *New York Times,* Section A, 20.

Ozonoff, S., Dawson, G., & McPartland, J. (2002). *A Parent's Guide to Asperger Syndrome and High-Functioning Autism.* Guilford Press, New York.

Ritvo, E. R., Freeman, B. J., Yuwiler, A., Geller, E., Yokota, A., Schroth, P., & Novak, P. (1984). Study of fenfluramine in outpatients with the syndrome of autism. *Journal of Pediatrics, 105,* 823–828.

Snyder, R., Turgay, A., Aman, M., Binder, C., Fisman, S., & Carroll, A. (2002). Effects of risperidone on conduct and disruptive behavior disorders in children with subaverage IQs. *Journal of the American Academy of Child and Adolescent Psychiatry, 41*(9), 1026–1036.

Unis, A. S., Munson, J. A., Rogers, S. J., Goldson, E., Osterling, J., Gabriels, R., Abbott, R. D., & Dawson, G. (2002). A randomized, double-blind, placebo-controlled trial of porcine versus synthetic secretin for reducing symptoms of autism. *Journal of the American Academy of Child and Adolescent Psychiatry, 41*(11), 1315–1321.

Volkmar, F. R. (1996). *Psychoses and Pervasive Developmental Disorder in Children and Adolescents.* American Psychiatric Press, Washington, DC.

Waltz, M. (2002). *Autistic Spectrum Disorders: Understanding the Diagnosis and Getting Help. Patient-Centered Guides* (2nd ed.). O'Reilly, Sebastopol, CA.

Yapko, D. (2003). *Understanding Autism Spectrum Disorders: Frequently Asked Questions.* Jessica Kingsley, London.

BIPOLAR DISORDER

Alessi, N., Naylor, M. W., Ghaziuddin, M., & Zubieta, J. K. (1994). Update on lithium carbonate therapy in children and adolescents. *Journal of the American Academy of Child and Adolescent Psychiatry, 33,* 291–304.

Biederman, J., Mick, E., Faraone, S. V., Spencer, T., Wilens, T. E., & Wozniak, J. (2000). Pediatric Mania: A developmental subtype of bipolar disorder? *Biological Psychiatry, 48*(6), 458–466.

DelBello, M. P., Kowatch, R. A., Warner, J., Schwiers, M. L., Rappaport, K. B., Daniels, J. P., Foster, K. D., & Strakowski, S. M. (2000). Adjunctive topiramate treatment for pediatric bipolar disorder: a retrospective chart review. *Journal of Child and Adolescent Psychopharmacology, 12(4), 323–330.*

Findling, R., Kowatch, R., & Post, R. (2003). *Pediatric Bipolar Disorder.* Martin Dunitz, London.

Frazier, J. A., Biederman, J., Tohen, M., Feldman, P. D., Jacobs, T. G., Toma, V., Rater, M. A., Tarazi, R. A., Kim, G. S., Garfield, S. B., Sohma, M., Gonzalez-Heydrich, J., Risser, R. C., & Nowlin, Z. M. (2001). A prospective open-label treatment trial of olanzapine monotherapy in children and adolescents with bipolar disorder. *Journal of Child and Adolescent Psychopharmacology, 11*(3), 239–250.

Geller, B., Cooper, T. B., Sun, K., Zimerman, B., Frazier, J., Williams, M., & Heath, J. (1998). Double-blind and placebo-controlled study of lithium for adolescent bipolar disorders with secondary substance dependency. *Journal of the American Academy of Child and Adolescent Psychiatry, 37*(2), 171–178.

Geller, B., Craney, J. L., Bolhofner, K., Nickelsburg, M. J., Williams, M., & Zimerman, B. (2002a). Two-year prospective follow-up of children with a prepubertal and early adolescent bipolar disorder phenotype. *American Journal of Psychiatry, 159,* 927–933.

Geller, B., Sun, K., Zimerman, B., Luby, J., Frazier, J., & Williams, M. (1995). Complex and rapid-cycling in bipolar children and adolescents: A preliminary study. *Journal of Affective Disorders, 34,* 1–10.

Geller, B., Zimerman, B., Williams, M., Delbello, M. P., Frazier, J., & Beringer, L. (2002b). Phenomenology of prepubertal and early adolescent bipolar disorder: Examples of elated mood, grandiose behaviors, decreased need for sleep, racing thoughts and hypersexuality. *Journal of Child and Adolescent Psychopharmacology, 12*(1), 3–9.

Kowatch, R. A., Suppes, T., Carmody, T. J., Bucci, J. P., Hume, J. H., Kromelis, M., Emslie, G. J., Weinberg, W. A., & Rush, A. J. (2000). Effect size of lithium, divalproex sodium, and carbamazepine in children and adolescents with bipolar disorder. *Journal of the American Academy of Child and Adolescent Psychiatry, 39*(6), 713–720.

McElroy, S., Strakowski, S., West, S., Keck, P., & McConville, B. (1997). Phenomenology of adolescent and adult mania in hospitalized patients with bipolar disorder. *American Journal of Psychiatry, 154,* 44–49.

Miklowitz, D. (2002). *The Bipolar Disorder Survival Guide: What You and Your Family Need to Know.* Guilford Press, New York.

Mondimore, F. M. (1999). *Bipolar Disorder: A Guide for Patients and Families.* John Hopkins University Press, Baltimore.

Papolos, D. (2002). *The Bipolar Child: The Definitive and Reassuring Guide to Childhood's Most Misunderstood Disorder* (rev. and exp. ed.). Broadway Books, New York.

Strober, M., Morrell, W., Lampert, C., & Burroughs, J. (1990). Relapse following discontinuation of lithium maintenance therapy in adolescents with bipolar I illness: A naturalistic study. *American Journal of Psychiatry, 147,* 457–461.

Weller, E. B., Weller, R. A., & Fristad, M. A. (1995). Bipolar disorder in children: Misdiagnosis, underdiagnosis, and future directions. *Journal of the American Academy of Child and Adolescent Psychiatry, 34,* 709–714.

Wilens, T. E., Biederman, J., Millstein, R., Wozniak, J., Hahesy, A., & Spencer, T. J. (1999). Risk for substance use disorders in youth with child- and adolescent-onset bipolar disorder. *Journal of the American Academy of Child and Adolescent Psychiatry, 38*(6), 680–685.

Wozniak, J., & Biederman, J. (1996). A pharmacological approach to the quagmire of comorbidity in juvenile mania. *Journal of the American Academy of Child and Adolescent Psychiatry, 35,* 826–829.

Wozniak, J., Biederman, J., Faraone, S. V., Frazier, J., Kim, J., Millstein, R., Gershon, J., Thornell, A., Cha, K., & Snyder, J. B. (1997). Mania in children with pervasive developmental disorder revisited. *Journal of the American Academy of Child & Adolescent Psychiatry, 36*(11), 1552–1559.

DEPRESSION

Bostic, J., & Wilens, T. (1997). Juvenile mood disorders and office psychopharmacology. *Adolescent Medicine, 44,* 1487–1503.

Birmaher, B., Brent, D. A., Kolko, D., Baugher, M., Bridge, J., Holder, D., Iyengar, S., & Ulloa, R. E. (2000). Clinical outcome after short-term psychotherapy for adolescents with major depressive disorder. *Archives of General Psychiatry, 57*(1), 29–36.

Brent, D. A., Baugher, M., Bridge, J., Chen, T., & Chiappetta, L. (1999). Age- and sex-related risk factors for adolescent suicide. *Journal of the American Academy of Child and Adolescent Psychiatry, 38*(12), 1497–1505.

Copeland, M. E. (2001). *Depression Workbook: A Guide to Living with Depression and Manic Depression* (2nd ed.). New Harbinger Publications, Oakland, CA.

Emslie, G. J., Rush, A. J., Weinberg, W. A., Kowatch, R. A., Hughes, C. W., Carmody, T., & Rintelmann, J. (1995). A double-blind, randomized, placebo-controlled trial of fluoxetine in children and adolescents with depression. *Archives of General Psychiatry, 54*(11), 1031–1037.

Emslie, G. J., Heiligenstein, J. H., Wagner, K. D., Hoog, S. L., Ernest, D. E., Brown, E., Nilsson, M., & Jacobson, J. G. (2002). Fluoxetine for acute treatment of depression in children and adolescents: a placebo-controlled, randomized clinical trial. *Journal of the American Academy of Child and Adolescent Psychiatry, 41*(10), 1205–1215.

Emslie, G. J., Rush, A. J., Weinberg, W. A., Kowatch, R. A., Hughes, C. W., Carmody, T., & Rintelmann, J. (1997). A double-blind, randomized, placebo-controlled trial of fluoxetine in children and adolescents with depression. *Archives of General Psychiatry, 54*(11), 1031–1037.

Goode, E. (2003, Dec. 11). British warning on antidepressant use for youth. *New York Times*, p. A1.

Gotlib, I. H., & Hammen, C. L., eds. (2002). *Handbook of Depression*. Guilford Press, New York.

Kovacs, M., Akiskal, H. S., Gatsonis, C., & Parrone, P. L. (1994). Childhood-onset dysthymic disorder: Clinical features and prospective naturalistic outcome. *Archives of General Psychiatry, 51*, 365–374.

Kovacs, M., Feinberg, T. L., Crouse-Novak, M. A., Paulauskas, S. L., & Finkelstein, R. (1984). Depressive disorders in childhood: I. A longitudinal prospective study of characteristics and recovery. *Archives of General Psychiatry, 41*, 229–237.

Kashani, J. H., & Sherman, D. D. (1989). Mood disorders in children and adolescents. In A. Tasman, R. E. Hales, and A. J. Frances, eds., *Review of Psychiatry* (pp. 197–217). American Psychiatric Press, Washington, DC.

Ryan, N. D., & Dahl, R. E. (1993). Neurobiology of depression in children and adolescents. *Clinical Neuroscience, 1*, 108–112.

Shafii, M., & Shafii, S. L. (1992). *Clinical Guide to Depression in Children and Adolescents*. American Psychiatric Press, Washington, DC.

Wagner, A., & Vitiello, B. (2002). Teen Angst from psychopathology. *Current Psychiatry, 1*(7), 41–50.

OBSESSIVE–COMPULSIVE DISORDER

Fitzgibbons, L., & Pedrick, C. (2003). *Helping Your Child with OCD: A Workbook for Parents of Children with Obsessive–Compulsive Disorder*. New Harbinger, Oakland, CA.

Francis, G. (1996) *Childhood Obsessive Compulsive Disorder.* Sage, Thousand Oaks, CA.

Geller, D. (2003). Special Issue on Obsessive Compulsive Disorder. *Journal of Child and Adolescent Psychopharmacology, 13*(suppl.).

Leonard, H. L., & Rapoport, J. L. (1989). Pharmacotherapy of childhood obsessive–compulsive disorder. In *Psychiatric Clinics of North America* (pp. 963–970). Saunders, Philadelphia.

March, J. S., Biederman, J., Wolkow, R., Safferman, A., Mardekian, J. Cook, E. H., et al. (1998). Sertraline in children and adolescents with obsessive–compulsive disorder: A multicenter randomized controlled trial. *Journal of the American Medical Association, 280,* 1752–1756.

Riddle, M. A., Reeve, E. A., Yaryura-Tobias, J. A., Yang, H. M., Claghorn, J. L., Gaffney, G., Greist, J. H., Holland, D., McConville, B. J., Pigott, T., & Walkup, J. T. (2001). Fluvoxamine for children and adolescents with obsessive–compulsive disorder: A randomized, controlled, multicenter trial. *Journal of the American Academy of Child and Adolescent Psychiatry, 40*(2), 222–229.

Rapoport, J. (1994). *The Boy Who Couldn't Stop Washing.* Dutton, New York.

Swedo, S. E., Leonard, H. L., Garvey, M., Mittleman, B., Allen, A. J., Perlmutter, S., Dow, S., Zamkoff, J., Dubbert, B. K., & Lougee, L. (1998). Pediatric autoimmune neuropsychiatric disorders asociated with streptococcal infections: Clinical description of the first 50 cases. *The American Journal of Psychiatry, 155*(2), 264–271.

Swedo, S. E., Rapoport, J. L., Leonard, H., Lenane, M., & Cheslow, D. (1989). Obsessive–compulsive disorder in children and adolescents. *Archives of General Psychiatry, 46,* 335–341.

Thomsen, P. H. (1999). *From Thoughts to Obsessions: Obsessive Compulsive Disorder in Children and Adolescents.* Jessica Kingsley, London.

Wagner, K. D., Cook, E. H., Chung, H., & Messig, M. (2003). Remission status after long-term Sertraline treatment of pediatric obsessive–compulsive disorder. *Journal of Child and Adolescent Psychopharmacology, 13*(suppl. 1), S53–S60.

PSYCHOSIS

Berke, J. (2001). *Beyond Madness: Psychosocial Interventions in Psychosis.* Jessica Kingsley, London.

Birchwood, M. J. (2001). *Early Intervention in Psychosis: A Guide to Concepts, Evidence and Interventions.* John Wiley, New York.

Boer, J. A., ed. (1996). *Advances in the Neurobiology of Schizophrenia.* John Wiley, New York.

Frazier, J. A., Spencer, T., Wilens, T., Wozniak, J., & Biederman, J. (1997). Childhood-onset schizophrenia, the prototypic disorder of childhood. *Psychiat-*

ric Clinics of North America: Annual Drug Therapy, 1997 (pp. 167–193). Saunders, Philadelphia.

Kumra, S., Jacobsen, L. K., Lenane, M., Karp, B. I., Frazier, J. A., Smith, A. K., Bedwell, J., Lee, P., Malanga, C. J., Hamburger, S., & Rapoport, J. L. (1998). Childhood-onset schizophrenia: An open-label study of olanzapine in adolescents. *Journal of the American Academy of Child and Adolescent Psychiatry, 37*(4), 377–385.

McClellan, J. M., & Werry, J. S. (1992). Schizophrenia. *Psychiatric Clinics of North America, 15,* 131–148.

Rapoport, J., Giedd, J., Blumenthal, J., Hamburger, S., Jeffries, N., Fernandez, T., Nicolson, R., Bedwell, J., Lenane, M., Zijdenbos, A., Paus, T., & Evans, A. (1999). Progressive cortical change during adolescence in childhood-onset schizophrenia. *Archives of General Psychiatry, 56*(7), 649–654.

Rapoport, J. L., Giedd, J., Kumra, S., Jacobsen, L., Smith, A., Lee, P., Nelson, J., & Hamburger, S. (1997). Childhood-onset schizophrenia. *Archives of General Psychiatry, 54,* 897–903.

Robbins, M. (1993). *Experiences of Schizophrenia: An Integration of the Personal, Scientific, and Therapeutic.* Guilford Press, New York.

Teicher, M., & Glod, C. (1990). Neuroleptic drugs: Indications and guidelines for their rational use in children and adolescents. *Journal of Child and Adolescent Psychopharmacology, 1,* 33–56.

Volkmar, F. R. (1996). *Psychoses and Pervasive Developmental Disorder in Children and Adolescence.* American Psychiatric Press, Washington, DC.

SUBSTANCE ABUSE

Bukstein, O. G., Brent, D. A., & Kaminer, Y. (1989). Comorbidity of substance abuse and other psychiatric disorders in adolescents. *American Journal of Psychiatry, 146,* 1131–1141.

Bukstein, O., Dunne, J. E., Arnold, V., Benson, R. S., Bernet, W., Kinlan, J., McClellan, J., & Sloan, L. E. (1998). Summary of the practice parameters for the assessment and treatment of children and adolescents with substance use disorders. *Journal of the American Academy of Child and Adolescent Psychiatry, 37*(1), 122–126.

Crowley, T. J., Macdonald, M. J., Whitmore, E. A., & Mikulich, S. K. (1998). Cannabis dependence, withdrawal, and reinforcing effects among adolescents with conduct symptoms and substance use disorders. *Drug and Alcohol Dependency, 50,* 27–37.

Galanter, M., ed. (1999). *American Psychiatric Press Textbook of Substance Abuse Treatment.* American Psychiatric Press, Arlington, VA.

Jaffee, S., ed. (1996). *Pediatric Substance Use Disorders (Vol. 1, Child and Adolescent Psychiatric Clinics of North America).* Saunders, Philadelphia.

Marlatt, A. (2002). *Harm Reduction Pragmatic Strategies for Managing High-Risk Behaviors.* Guilford Press, New York.

Riggs, P. D., & Davies, R. D. (2002). A clinical approach to integrating treatment for adolescent depression and substance abuse. *Journal of the American Academy of Child and Adolescent Psychiatry, 41*(10), 1253–1255.

Riggs, P. D. (1998). Clinical approach to treatment of ADHD in adolescents with substance use disorders and conduct disorder. *Journal of the American Academy of Child and Adolescent Psychiatry, 37*(3), 331–332.

Volpicelli, J. (2000). *Recovery Options: The Complete Guide.* John Wiley, New York.

Waldron, H. B., Slesnick, N., Bordy, J., Turner, C. W., & Peterson, T. R. (2001). Treatment outcomes for adolescent substance abuse at 4- and 7- month assessments. *Journal of Consulting and Clinical Psychology, 69,* 802–813.

Waxmonsky, J., & Wilens, T. (2003). Substance abusing youths. In A. Martin, L. Scahill, D. S. Charney, & J. F. Leckman, eds., *Pediatric Psychopharmacology: Principles and Practice* (pp. 605–616). Oxford University Press, New York.

TIC AND TOURETTE'S DISORDER

Chappell, P., Riddle, M., Scahill, L., Lynch, K., Schultz, R., Arnsten, A., Leckman, J., & Cohen, D. (1995). Guanfacine treatment of comorbid attention-deficit hyperactivity hyperactivity disorder and Tourette's syndrome. *Journal of the American Academy of Child and Adolescent Psychiatry, 34,* 1140–1146.

Cohen, D. J., Detlor, J., Young, J. G., & Shaywitz, B. A. (1980). Clonidine ameliorates Gilles de la Tourette's syndrome. *Archives of General Psychiatry, 37,* 1350–1357.

Cohen, D. J., Bruun, R. D., & Leckman, J. F., eds. (1988). *Tourette's Syndrome and Tic Disorders: Clinical Understanding and Treatment.* John Wiley, New York.

Haerle, T. (2003). *Children With Tourette Syndrome: A Parent's Guide.* Woodbine House, Bethesda, MD.

Kurlan, R. (2002). Treatment of ADHD in children with tics: A randomized controlled trial. *Neurology, 58,* 527–536.

Leckman, J. (2001). *Tourette's Syndrome: Tics, Obsessions, Compulsions: Developmental Psychopathology and Clinical Care.* John Wiley, New York.

Leckman, J. F., Hardin, M. T., Riddle, M. A., Stevenson, J., Ort, S. I., & Cohen, D. J. (1991). Clonidine treatment of Gilles de la Tourette's syndrome. *Archives of General Psychiatry, 48,* 324–328.

Robertson, M. (1998) *Tourette Syndrome: The Facts.* Oxford University Press, London; New York.

Scahill, L. (2001). Controlled clinical trial of guanfacine in ADHD youth with tic disorders. *American Journal of Psychiatry, 158,* 1067–1074.

Spencer, T., Biederman, J., Coffey, B., Geller, D., Wilens, T., & Faraone, S.

(1999). The 4-year course of tic disorders in boys with attention-deficit/hyperactivity disorder. *Archives of General Psychiatry, 56,* 842–847.

MISCELLANEOUS

Chokroverty, S. (2001). *100 Questions about Sleep and Sleep Disorders.* Blackwell, Malden, MA.

Costin, C. (1999). *The Eating Disorder Sourcebook: A Comprehensive Guide to the Causes, Treatments, and Prevention of Eating Disorders.* McGraw-Hill, New York.

Dahl, R. E., & Puig-Antich, J. (1990). Sleep disturbances in child and adolescent psychiatric disorders, *Pediatrician, 17,* 32–37.

Fairburn, C. G., & Brownell, K. D. (2001) *Eating Disorders and Obesity: A Comprehensive Handbook.* Guilford Press, New York.

Jimmerson, D. C., Herzog, D. B., & Brotman, A. W. (1993). Pharmacological approaches in the treatment of eating disorders. *Harvard Review of Psychiatry, 1,* 82–93.

Loney, J. (1988). Substance abuse in adolescents: Diagnostic issues derived from studies of attention deficit disorder with hyperactivity. *NIDA Research Monograph, 77,* 19–26.

Palm, L., Blennow, G., & Wetterberg, L. (1997). Long-term melatonin treatment in blind children and young adults with circadian sleep-wake disturbances. *Developmental Medicine and Child Neurology, 39,* 319–325.

Prince, J., Wilens, T., Biederman, J., Spencer, T., & Wozniak, J. (1996). Clonidine for sleep disturbances associated with attention-deficit hyperactivity disorder: A systematic chart review of 62 cases. *Journal of the American Academy of Child and Adolescent Psychiatry, 35*(5), 599–605.

Reite, M. (1997) *Concise Guide to Evaluation and Management of Sleep Disorders* (2nd ed.). American Psychiatric Press, Arlington, VA.

Robins, L. N. (1966). *Deviant Children Grown Up.* Williams & Wilkins, Baltimore.

Thompson, K. J., ed. (2001). *Body Image, Eating Disorders, and Obesity in Youth: Assessment, Prevention, and Treatment.* American Psychological Association, Washington, DC.

INDEX

ABOUT THE AUTHOR

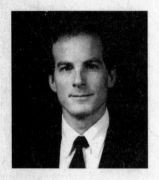

Timothy E. Wilens, MD, is Associate Professor of Psychiatry at Harvard Medical School and Director of Substance Abuse Services in the Pediatric Psychopharmacology Clinic at Massachusetts General Hospital. Board-certified in child, adolescent, adult, and addiction psychiatry, Dr. Wilens specializes in pediatric and adult psychopharmacology. He earned his MD at the University of Michigan Medical School and completed his residency at Massachusetts General Hospital under the auspices of Harvard Medical School.

Dr. Wilens' research interests include the relationship between attention-deficit/hyperactivity disorder (ADHD), bipolar disorder, and substance abuse; the pharmacotherapy of ADHD across the lifespan; and juvenile bipolar disorder. He is the author of more than 55 book chapters, 140 scientific articles in peer-reviewed journals, and 180 abstracts and presentations for national and international scientific meetings. A Distinguished Fellow of the American Psychiatric Association and the American Academy of Child and Adolescent Psychiatry, among many other professional societies, Dr. Wilens is consistently named among the Best of Boston—Child/Adult Psychiatry and the Top/Best Doctors in America.